Promoting Health

A Practical Guide

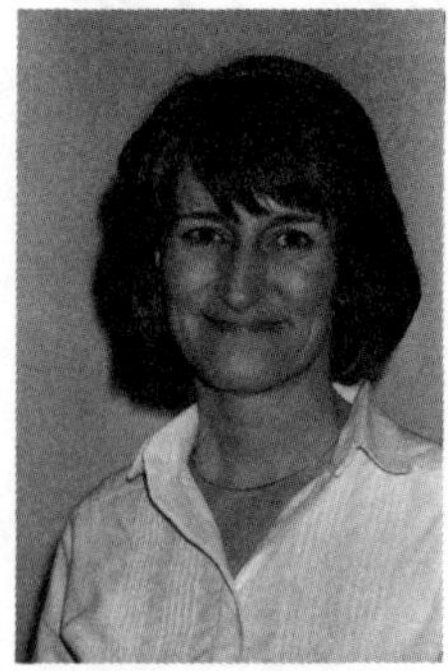

Linda Ewles *MSc BSc SRD*

Linda Ewles became the Purchasing Manager for Health Promotion in Bristol & District Health Authority in 1991, responsible for developing the health promotion perspective on health needs, policy development and contracts for health promotion services and programmes. She began her career as a dietitian, and worked in hospital and community dietetics in England and Bermuda. She then moved into health education as a health education officer in East Sussex for several years. Afterwards came five years as Senior Lecturer in Health Education at Bristol Polytechnic, where she directed the postgraduate Diploma in Health Education, the recognised qualification for health education officers. She also taught health education, nutrition and communication to students on health visiting, district nursing, community psychiatric and mental handicap nursing and nursing degree courses. Linda then moved from teaching to practice as the District Health Promotion Officer for Bristol & Weston Health Authority for six years. During this time, as head of the district's growing Health Promotion Department, she gained much practical experience of planning and managing health promotion, often in collaboration with a range of statutory and voluntary agencies. She was also actively involved in planning and teaching health promotion on in-service training courses for health and allied professionals, participating in national and local conferences and serving on professional associations and advisory bodies on health promotion.

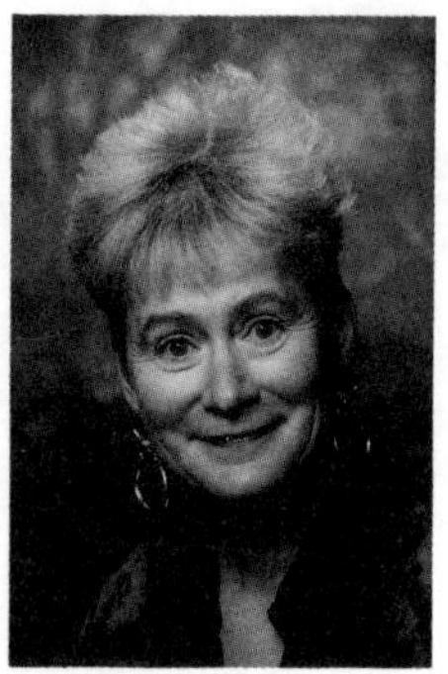

Ina Simnett *MA(Oxon) DPhil CertEd*

Ina Simnett works as a freelance trainer and consultant. Her current activities include running an Open Learning Centre for Health Service managers and writing open learning materials. She is a contributor and consultant to the Certificate in Health Education Open Learning Project at Keele University. She began her career as a research physiologist, then worked as an adult education tutor and freelance broadcaster while bringing up her three daughters. Following teacher training and a period as a biology teacher and sixth-form tutor, she worked in health education for twelve years as Area Health Education Officer for Northumberland Area Health Authority and for a further period as Regional Coordinator for the Health Education Council's 'Understanding Alcohol' Programme in South-west England. More recently she has worked as a Training Consultant with the National Health Service Training Authority and as a management trainer. Ina has extensive experience of teaching health promotion to health professionals, teachers and social services staff. She has contributed to a number of open learning packages and training manuals and has recently written a package *Promoting Health: Local Authorities in Action* for the Health Education Authority. She is committed to playing an active role in the development of women—including herself—and runs workshops on promoting sexual health for women.

Promoting Health:

A Practical Guide

Second Edition

Linda Ewles MSc BSc SRD

Ina Simnett MA(Oxon) DPhil CertEd

Scutari Press. London

Scutari Press is a division of Scutari Projects Ltd,
the publishing company of the Royal College of Nursing.

This edition is first published in 1992.
Reprinted 1992

British Library Cataloguing in Publication Data:

Ewles, Linda
Promoting health: A practical guide.—2nd ed.
I. Title II. Simnett, Ina
613
ISBN 1-871364-73-6

Printed in Great Britain at the Alden Press, Oxford

To all those working to reduce inequalities in health

Contents

Preface ... xi

Acknowledgements ... xii

Note on Terminology ... xii

Introduction ... xiii

PART I: THINKING ABOUT HEALTH AND HEALTH PROMOTION

Chapter 1 **Concepts and Determinants of Health** ... 3

What Does 'Being Healthy' Mean to You? ... 3
Lay and Professional Concepts of Health ... 4
Towards a Holistic Concept of Health ... 6
What Affects Health? ... 9
Addressing the Determinants of Health ... 12
Notes, References and Further Reading ... 14

Chapter 2 **What is Health Promotion?** ... 19

Defining Health Promotion ... 19
Health Promotion or Health Education? ... 20
The Scope of Health Promotion ... 20
A Framework for Health Promotion Activities ... 25
Developing Competence in Health Promotion ... 27
Notes, References and Further Reading ... 29

Chapter 3 **Philosophical Issues in Health Promotion** ... 32

Clarifying Health Promotion Aims ... 32
Analysing Your Aims and Values: Five Approaches ... 35
Some More Ethical Dilemmas ... 38
Making Ethical Decisions ... 42
Towards a Code of Practice... 44
Notes, References and Further Reading ... 45

Chapter 4 **Identifying Health Promoters and Their Roles** 48

Agents and Agencies of Health Promotion 48
Improving Your Health Promotion Role 57
Notes, References and Further Reading 58

PART II: MOVING FROM THEORY TO PRACTICE

Chapter 5 **Identifying Health Promotion Needs and Priorities** 67

Concepts of Need 68
Identifying Health Promotion Needs 70
Finding and Using Information 72
Assessing Health Promotion Needs 75
Setting Health Promotion Priorities 78
Notes, References and Further Reading 80

Chapter 6 **Planning and Evaluating** 84

The Planning and Evaluation Process 84
Stage 1: Identify Needs and Priorities 86
Stage 2: Set Aims and Objectives 86
Stage 3: Decide the Best Way of Achieving the Aims 90
Stage 4: Identify Resources 92
Stage 5: Plan Evaluation Methods 94
Stage 6: Set an Action Plan 98
Stage 7: Action! 99
Notes, References and Further Reading 100

Chapter 7 **Some Key Aspects of Managing Health Promotion** 103

Working with Other People: Co-ordination and Teamwork 104
Working with Other People: Participating in Meetings 106
Working with Other People: Effective Committee Work 107
Communicating with Colleagues: Analysing your Communication Channels 110
Communicating with Colleagues: Writing Reports 111
Managing Paperwork: Information Systems 113
Managing Time 113
Notes, References and Further Reading 116

PART III: DEVELOPING COMPETENCE IN HEALTH PROMOTION

Chapter 8 **Fundamentals of Communication** 121

Exploring Relationships with Clients 121
Communication Barriers 124
Overcoming Language Barriers 126

Non-verbal Communication ... 127
Listening ... 131
Helping People to Talk... 132
Asking Questions and Getting Feedback... 134
Notes, References and Further Reading ... 137

Chapter 9 **Working with Groups** ... 139

Kinds of Groups ... 140
Group Leadership ... 140
Group Behaviour ... 144
Setting up a Group ... 146
Getting Groups Going ... 148
Discussion Skills ... 150
Dealing with Difficulties ... 153
Notes, References and Further Reading ... 155

Chapter 10 **Helping People to Make Health Choices** ... 158

Working for Client Self-empowerment ... 159
Strategies for Increasing Self-awareness, Clarifying Values and Changing Attitudes ... 159
Strategies for Decision-making ... 164
Strategies for Changing Behaviour ... 166
Using Strategies Effectively... 170
Notes, References and Further Reading ... 172

Chapter 11 **Teaching and Instructing** ... 175

What Makes a Good Teacher? ... 175
Some Principles of Effective Teaching ... 176
Guidelines for Giving Talks ... 180
Improved Patient Education ... 183
Teaching Practical Skills ... 186
Notes, References and Further Reading ... 186

Chapter 12 **Working with Communities** ... 190

Community-based Work in Health Promotion ... 190
Key Terms ... 191
Principles of Community-based Work ... 192
Community Participation ... 193
Community Development ... 196
Community Health Projects ... 199
Developing Competences in Community Work ... 204
Notes, References and Further Reading ... 205

Chapter 13 **Changing Policy and Practice** ... 208

Who Makes Health Policies? ... 209
Challenging Health-damaging Policy ... 210
Characteristics of Power and Influence ... 211
The Politics of Influence ... 212
Developing and Implementing Policies ... 215
Campaigning ... 219
Implementing Change ... 220
Notes, References and Further Reading ... 222

Chapter 14 **Using and Producing Health Promotion Materials** ... 226

Health Promotion Materials: Criteria for Choice ... 226
The Range of Materials—Uses, Advantages and Limitations ... 228
Producing Materials ... 232
Presenting Statistical Information ... 238
Notes, References and Further Reading ... 241

Chapter 15 **Working with the Mass Media** ... 243

Mass Media as Channels for Health Issues ... 243
Using the Mass Media for Health Promotion ... 244
Working with Radio and Television ... 248
Working with the Local Press ... 251
Notes, References and Further Reading ... 256

Index ... 259

Preface

The aim of this book is to provide an easy-to-read, practical guide for all those who practise health promotion in their everyday work. The people we refer to include health professionals such as health education/promotion officers, hospital and community nurses, health visitors and midwives, hospital doctors and general practitioners, dentists and dental hygienists, health service managers and the professions allied to medicine, for example dietitians and chiropodists. We also include a very wide range of statutory and non-statutory agents and agencies, for example local authority staff (such as environmental health officers planners, housing officers and social services staff), voluntary organisations, charities, pressure groups and self-help groups, youth and community workers, and teachers in schools, colleges and institutions of higher education, probation officers and police officers. For all these people, whether they are students in basic or postbasic training, or individuals with years of experience who wish to take a fresh look at the health promotion aspects of their work, this book will encourage the establishment of sound principles on which to base their own practice and improve their competence in a variety of health promotion methods.

The book is designed to be used as a self-teaching aid and as a source of material and ideas for group teaching for course tutors. We have included exercises, case studies, quizzes, questionnaires and cartoons to make learning stimulating, relevant and enjoyable.

The first edition of this book was welcomed by students and tutors on many courses, such as courses for training health visitors, teachers and district nurses, postgraduate courses in health education and health promotion, Health Education Certificate courses, and by many other health promoters, for three main reasons. One is that health promotion is an applied field of study rather than an established discipline in its own right. As a result, it is difficult for health promoters to locate relevant and understandable material, which is scattered throughout a wide range of sources. Secondly, health promotion is receiving greater emphasis in the training and practice of an ever-widening range of disciplines and professions. Thirdly, the general public is increasingly interested in health issues, and is expressing a need for more health promotion.

Since the publication of the first edition, the evolution of health promotion has accelerated, and we have produced the second edition in response to the need expressed by many health promoters, who are eagerly awaiting its publication. We hope that this edition will be useful both to those who have used the first edition, and to the increasing number of people who are becoming actively involved in improving the health status of the population, through empowering themselves and others to take more control over aspects of their lives which affect their health. We hope that this book will challenge, inform and contribute to the spread of good practice in health promotion.

Acknowledgements

We are indebted to numerous people who have shared with us their health promotion experience and ideas. They include tutors and students on courses such as Health Education Diploma and Certificate courses, basic training courses for a range of health professionals, and professional development courses for teachers, youth workers, environmental health officers, police, social services staff and others. Wherever possible, the exercises contained in the book have been tested with one or more of these groups of students, and without their involvement it would have been impossible to produce a book which is, we hope, relevant to the real needs and concerns of all health promoters.

We would also like to acknowledge the contribution of all those people who have influenced the development of our own learning and ideas. Special thanks are due to Stella Mountford, Keith Hazeltine, Alan Beattie, Sue Habeshaw, Trevor Habeshaw, Stewart Greenwell, Roger Silver, Jane Randell, John Heron, Hazel Johns, Donna Brandes, Bob Ticktum, Martin Evans, Linda Wright, Peter Allen, Ian Fairfax and all the health promotion officers in the Bristol & Weston Health Promotion Department.

We are grateful to many people for giving us ideas for exercises included in this book, but especially to Sue Habeshaw and Penny Mares.

We would like to thank Peter England, Iain Harkess, Sue Steel and Kathy Weare for reading draft chapters and offering support and critical comment. Students on the Health Education Certificate Course at Brunel Technical College, Bristol, 1989/90 and 1990/91 and the MA in health education at Southampton University 1990/91 have been particularly helpful with comments, new teaching ideas and exercises and as fruitful sources of case students and illustrative examples.

Many other people have helped in different ways. We appreciate and thank Jan Smithies for producing the foundation material for Chapter 12 *Working with Communities*, Christopher Flook for ideas and skill in producing the cartoons, and Ian Baker and Clive Baish for support.

Finally, for their practical and moral support we thank our partners, Jack Humphreys and Jim Pimpernell, and our editor, Patrick West.

Note on Terminology

We have tried to practise non-sexist writing throughout this book, using the principles and ideas we discuss in the paragraphs on non-sexist writing in Chapter 14. We have not always succeeded, and there are times when, for the sake of clarity, we have needed to refer to a health promoter or a client as ‘he’ or ‘she’. In these instances, we have chosen to refer to the health promoter as ‘she’, and to the recipient of health promotion as ‘he’. This is not, of course, intended to imply that all health promoters are female, nor that people receiving or using health promotion are always male. It is simply to avoid confusion and clumsy repetition of ‘he/she’ and ‘himself/herself’.

Also, we have often referred to the people health promoters are working with as ‘patients’, ‘consumers’, ‘users’ or ‘clients’. This does not imply, for example, that where we have referred to patients the text is irrelevant to healthy clients or vice-versa. It is solely to avoid the use of awkward terms such as ‘patient or client’.

Introduction to the Second Edition

This book is addressed to all health promoters—everyone who practises health promotion as all or part of their everyday work.

Health promotion in the UK today encompasses a wide variety of activities with the common purpose of improving the health status of individuals and communities. This book is concerned with the *what*, *why*, *who* and *how* of health promotion. It aims to help to explore important questions such as:

- What is health?
- What affects health?
- What is health promotion and what is health education?
- Who are the agents and agencies of health promotion?
- Who needs health promotion and what are these needs?
- How can health promotion be planned, managed and evaluated? How can priorities be set?
- How can health promoters best carry out health promotion? What are the competences they require?
- What are the key issues currently facing health promotion?

The range of health 'topics' is clearly enormous, and different professions and disciplines will all have their own areas of expert knowledge. They will also have specialist skills, for example in treatment, therapy or technical tests. We do not aim to discuss these topics or specialist areas of knowledge and skills, but to focus on the theories, principles and competences which you need to consider whatever your background.

As in the first edition, we have organised the book into three sections. *Part I: Thinking about Health and Health Promotion* deals with basic ideas of what health, health promotion and health education are about, the different approaches and ethical issues which need to be considered, and identifies the agencies and people who have a part to play in promoting health.

Part II: Moving from Theory to Practice looks at how you can decide on needs and priorities, plan, evaluate and manage your work.

Part III: Developing Competence in Health Promotion looks at how you can develop your competence in carrying out a range of activities including teaching, group work, helping people to make health choices, working with communities, changing policies and practices, and working with the mass media. The fundamentals of communication and of using and producing health promotion materials are also addressed.

Since the publication of the first edition, there have been a number of important changes which we have taken account of in this edition.

First, health education has become subsumed in a broader approach to promoting health, encompassing both efforts to change socioeconomic and environmental conditions and health education aimed at individuals, groups and communities. This has been called the 'new public health movement'. It is characterised by renewed efforts of statutory and non-statutory agencies, working collaboratively to improve the health of individuals and communities. The second edition reflects these developments by addressing a wider range of people and discussing broader approaches and methods.

Secondly, the World Health Organisation, the UK government and other significant organisations have emphasised the importance of agreeing targets for health promotion, both nationally and locally. As a result, an increasing number of cities, towns and communities are now working towards agreed targets, and have adopted a strategic approach to health promotion. This has been accompanied by an increased emphasis on the management, planning and evaluation of health promotion. Part Two of the second edition reflects these changes.

Part Three follows through, with an emphasis on developing competence in health promotion, as an important contribution to quality assurance. We address the core competences needed to practise health promotion. These include not only traditional health education competences in communicating and educating, but also in managing, researching, planning, evaluating, marketing, facilitating, networking and influencing policies and practices.

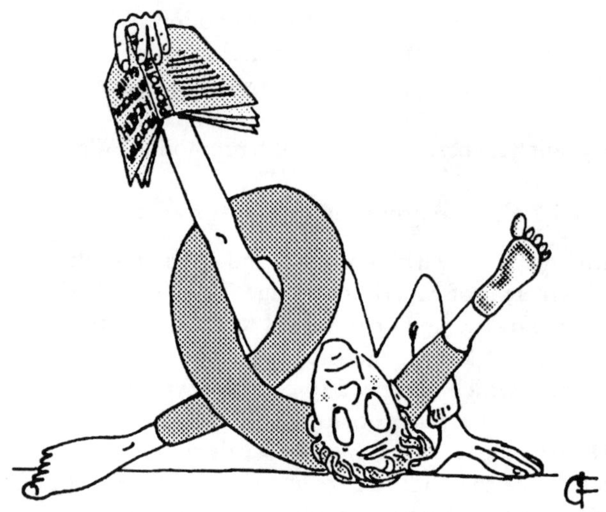

Studying this book will be an active educational experience

Third, health promoters are accountable to the communities they serve. More attention is being paid to the views of users and receivers of health promotion, and to the concept of working in partnership with the public. Ways to encourage the active participation of individuals, groups and communities in planning, implementing and evaluating health promotion are emphasised throughout this edition. The way to improve health is through personal and community empowerment, so that people can have more control over aspects of their lives which affect their health.

Fourthly, this edition has been updated to take account of the major changes in the way national and local services are organised and delivered. New legislation, such as the 1990 NHS and Community Care Act, will bring further changes, and we take account of the likely impact on health promotion. More emphasis is also placed on international developments such as the emerging influence of the European Community.

Finally, this edition takes account of global factors, such as the importance of the environment and ecosystems for human health and well-being.

We have retained the broad aims and 'user-friendly' approach adopted in the first edition. We aim to keep you involved, so that studying this book will be an active educational experience.

We have included exercises to do as an individual or in a group, and examples and case studies which we hope will help you to apply ideas to your own situation. Often the exercises are designed to stimulate thought and discussion, and as there may be no 'right' answers, we do not provide them. Some readers may find this frustrating or uncomfortable: if so, we ask you to think it through, talk it over and work it out for yourself. In this way the 'answers' will have personal meaning and application. This is an example of how education can play a part in personal empowerment, and models the sort of approach we advocate in health promotion.

PART I

THINKING ABOUT HEALTH AND HEALTH PROMOTION

Introduction

Part I has three purposes.

- It sets the context for the whole book by introducing key concepts, principles and ideas, and providing you with a shared language in which to communicate about health promotion.
- It provides an introduction to the dimensions and scope of health and health promotion, which enables you to focus on the wide range of activities and approaches and on the diverse agents and agencies involved.
- It highlights important philosophical and ethical issues which are explored in a practical context later in the book.

Health is an extremely difficult word to define but it is clearly important that you know what it is that you are promoting. This is discussed in Chapter One, along with a description of the major influences on health and the origins of inequalities in health.

Chapter Two explores the scope of health promotion and demonstrates that it encompasses a wide range of activities. A framework for classifying the major areas of health promotion activity is offered, and the competences which you need in order to practise health promotion are identified.

Chapter Three analyses the aims and values associated with different approaches to health promotion, explores a number of ethical dilemmas, and provides guidance on how to make ethical decisions.

Chapter Four identifies the agents and agencies of health promotion and provides you with help in clarifying your own health promotion role.

Chapter 1
Concepts and Determinants of Health

Summary

This chapter begins by looking at what 'being healthy' means to the reader and then reviews the wide variation in people's concepts of health. The next section identifies dimensions of health (physical, mental, emotional, social, spiritual and societal) and discusses a holistic concept. This leads on to identifying and examining factors which affect health, including a discussion of the role of medicine and the issue of widening inequalities in health. The final section looks at how the fundamental determinants of health are being addressed, and reviews the 'health for all' and 'new public health' movements.

What Does 'Being Healthy' Mean to You?

'Being healthy' means different things to different people. Much has been researched and written about people's varying concepts of health, and references are given at the end of this chapter for the interested reader.[1] More important than academic discussion, though, is the need for all health promoters to explore and define for yourselves what being healthy means to you and may mean to your clients.

Exercise — What does 'being healthy' mean to you?[2]

In Column 1, tick any of the statements which seem to you to be important aspects of your health. Tick as many as you like.

For me, being healthy involves:	Column 1	Column 2	Column 3
1. Enjoying being with my family and friends	______	______	______
2. Living to a ripe old age	______	______	______
3. Feeling happy most of the time	______	______	______

continued on next page

continued

4. Having a job	______	______	______
5. Hardly ever taking tablets or medicines	______	______	______
6. Being the ideal weight for my height	______	______	______
7. Taking regular exercise	______	______	______
8. Feeling at peace with myself	______	______	______
9. Never smoking	______	______	______
10. Never suffering from anything more serious than a mild cold, flu or stomach upset	______	______	______
11. Not getting things confused or out of proportion—assessing situations realistically	______	______	______
12. Being able to adapt easily to big changes in my life such as moving house or a new job	______	______	______
13. Drinking only moderate amounts of alcohol or none at all	______	______	______
14. Enjoying my work without too much stress	______	______	______
15. Having all the parts of my body in good working condition	______	______	______
16. Getting on well with other people most of the time	______	______	______
17. Eating the 'right' foods	______	______	______
18. Enjoying some form of relaxation or recreation	______	______	______

In Column 2, tick the six statements which are the *most important* aspects of 'being healthy' to you.

Then in Column 3, rank these six in the order of importance—put 1 by the most important, 2 by the next most important and so on down to 6.

If you are working in a group, compare your list with other people's. Look at the similarities and differences, and discuss the reasons for your choices.

Lay and Professional Concepts of Health

To the general public, being healthy may just mean 'not being ill'. Health is taken for granted, only considered when illness or health problems are interfering with people's everyday lives. This may be summed up as 'you don't think about your health until you've lost it'.

There are, perhaps, some more positive ways in which the general public thinks of health. The first is reflected in phrases like 'building up strength' and having 'resistance' to infection. This implies that health means strength and robustness, and having reserves which can be called on to fight illness and cope with stress and fatigue. Secondly, people talk about being 'off-colour' or 'out of sorts' or, conversely, being 'in good form'. In this way, health may be closely associated with moods and feelings, and a sense of balance and equilibrium.[3]

Researchers in different settings have found a wealth of complex notions about health. For example, mothers of families with small children in Wales specified that having the capacity to cope and function as expected was an important aspect of 'health' for them, and they also associated positive health with being cheerful and enthusiastic.[4] Other researchers have found that people see health and illness as moral categories: some socially-disadvantaged women in a Scottish study thought of illness in terms of spiritual or moral malaise.[5] Elderly Scottish people saw three major dimensions of health; the absence of illness and disease, a dimension of strength–weakness, and being fit to do the jobs expected.[6]

Concepts of health are linked with people's social and cultural situations. Thus, to the mothers of small children in the Welsh study, coping with the family was their key concern. Middle-class women are more likely to identify aspects of emotional or mental well-being as part of their idea of health than working-class women, who more frequently concentrate on being physically fit.[7] 'Folk knowledge' of illness, prevention and treatment can also be powerful in shaping people's concept of health. Such knowledge may be part of a cultural heritage, passed on through generations.[8]

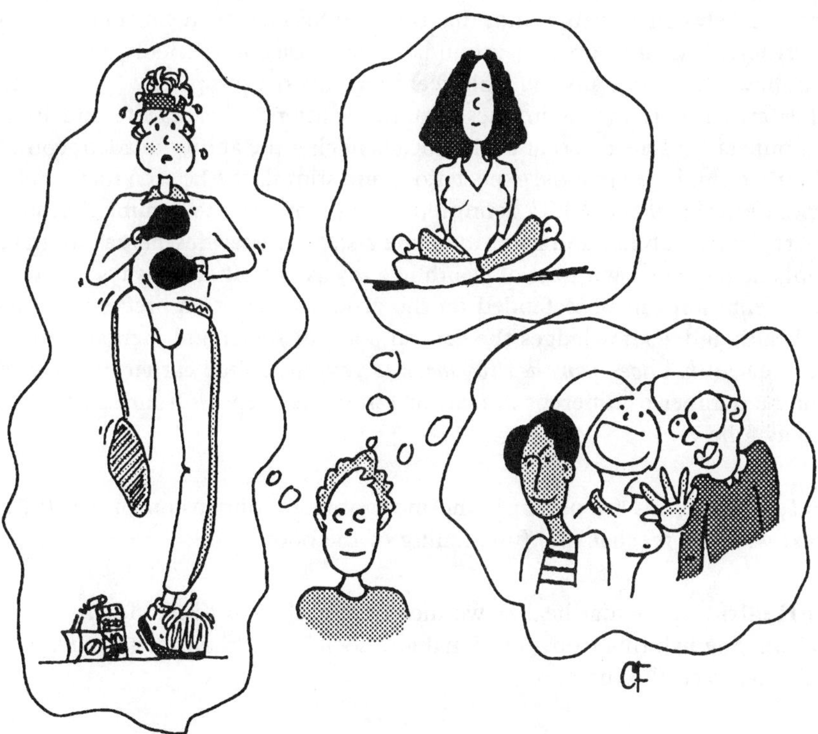

People's ideas of 'being healthy' vary widely

Standards of what may be considered 'healthy' also vary. An elderly person may say she is in good health on a day when her chronic bronchitis and arthritis have eased up enough to enable her to hobble down to the shops. A smoker may not report his early-morning cough as a symptom of ill-health, because to him it is normal. People assess their own health subjectively, according to their own norms and expectations. This is one of the reasons why attempts to measure health (as opposed to measuring illness) are especially difficult.[9]

To summarise, then, people's ideas of 'health' and 'being healthy' vary widely. They are shaped by their experiences, knowledge, values and expectations, as well as their view of what they are expected to do in their everyday lives, and the fitness they need to fulfil that role.

To professionals in the field, 'health' may be viewed more objectively as freedom from medically-defined disease and disability. But there may be a world of difference between a lay and a professional person's perception of what 'counts' as illness or disability, what causes it and what to do about it.[10]

Towards a Holistic Concept of Health

Several decades ago, the World Health Organisation (WHO) defined health as 'a state of complete physical, mental and social well-being, and not merely the absence of disease and infirmity'.[11] This statement is still extensively quoted, although WHO has developed its view considerably since that time.[12] This historic definition has also been heavily criticised, mainly on two grounds. One is that it is totally unrealistic and idealistic (how often does anyone truly feel in a state of 'complete . . . well-being'?). The other criticism is that it implies a static position, whereas life and living are anything but static. The idea that health means having the ability to adapt continually to constantly changing demands, expectations and stimuli can be seen to be preferable.

Another criticism of the WHO definition is that it appears to assume that someone, somewhere, has the ability and right to define a state of health, whereas we have seen that people define their own state of health in a myriad of different ways. On the other hand, the definition can be defended on the grounds that it embraces the notion of positive health and acknowledges the central place of social and mental well-being.

The exercise *What does being healthy mean to you*? described earlier, involves you in identifying a number of different dimensions in the concept of health. These may be classified as follows.

Physical Health: this is, perhaps, the most obvious dimension of health, and is concerned with the mechanistic functioning of the body.

Mental Health: by mental health, we mean the ability to think clearly and coherently. We distinguish this from emotional and social health, although there is a close association between the three.

Emotional Health: this means the ability to recognise emotions such as fear, joy, grief and anger and to express such emotions appropriately. Emotional or 'affective' health also means coping with stress, tension, depression and anxiety.

Social Health: social health means the ability to make and maintain relationships with other people.

Spiritual Health: this, for some people, is connected with religious beliefs and practices; for other people it is to do with personal creeds, principles of behaviour and ways of achieving peace of mind and being at peace with oneself.

Societal Health: so far, we have considered health at the level of the individual, but a person's health is inextricably related to everything surrounding that person. It is impossible to be healthy in a 'sick' society which does not provide the resources for basic physical and emotional needs. For example, people obviously cannot be healthy if they cannot afford necessities for food, clothing and shelter, but nor can they be healthy in countries of extreme political oppression where basic human rights are denied. Women cannot be healthy when their contribution to society is undervalued, and neither black nor white can be healthy in a racist society where racism undermines human worth, self-esteem and social relationships. Unemployed people cannot be healthy in a society which only values people in paid employment, and it is very unlikely that anyone can be healthy if they live in an area which lacks basic services and facilities such as health care, transport and recreation. Michael Wilson puts this graphically when he says that health cannot be possessed, 'It can only be shared. There is no health for me without my brother. There is no health for Britain without Bangladesh.'[13]

The Holistic View

The identification of these different aspects of health is a useful exercise in raising awareness of the complexity of the concept of health. But in practice, it is obvious that dividing people's lives into 'physical', 'mental' and so on often imposes artificial divisions and unhelpful distortions of a situation. Sexual health, for example, crosses all these boundaries. All aspects of health are interrelated and interdependent, and we subscribe to the view that a holistic view of health is of greater value to you and the people you work with.

Case study—Dimensions of health

Bob smokes 20 cigarettes a day and is prone to bronchitis each winter. He knows that smoking causes him to cough in the mornings, aggravates his bronchitis and is making it more likely that he will develop heart disease, which killed his father. He continues to smoke because it is the only way he finds he can cope with the demands of his job. When he tries to stop smoking he feels so tense and irritable that his work suffers and he becomes very bad-tempered with his wife and child. For Bob, his emotional and social health depend on his smoking, and this outweighs the disadvantages to his physical health. He thinks that the only way he could stop smoking is to find a less pressured job.

Exercise—Dimensions of health

1. Go back to your answers in the previous exercise *What does being healthy mean to you?*

Tick any of the following dimensions of health that are reflected in the statements you ticked in Column 1:

physical ______
mental ______
social ______
emotional ______
spiritual ______
societal ______

Is any one of these dimensions more important to you than the others? How do they relate to each other?

2. Has your idea of 'health' changed since childhood? If so, how and why? How do you think a child's concept of health differs from an adult's?

3. If you have had professional training in health or a related area of work, what difference do you think this has made to your idea of health?

4. What do you think 'being healthy' may mean to someone who:
   - is mentally handicapped?
   - has a permanent physical disability such as deafness or paralysis?
   - has an illness or infection for which there is currently no known cure such as diabetes, arthritis, HIV, schizophrenia?
   - lives below the poverty line?

5. Identify three or four key points you have learnt from this exercise about your own ideas of 'being healthy'.

Other writers have provided useful analyses of what 'health' means from the viewpoint of a philosopher and a sociologist, and these are recommended for further study.[14] One of these (Seedhouse) proposes the idea of health as the foundation for achieving a person's realistic potential: enabling people to fulfil their own potential. It is about *empowering* people: enabling them to become all that they are capable of becoming.[15] Working for health is thus linked closely with improving people's *quality of life*.

This notion of *health as the foundations for achieving human potential* has much to offer the health worker. It recognises that health is a dynamic state, that each person's potential is different, that each person's health needs are different. Working for health is both an individual and a societal responsibility, and involves empowering people to improve their quality of life.

WHO also identify key aspects of 'health' which encompass these notions. WHO propose:

> . . . a conception of health as the extent to which an individual or group is able, on the one hand, to realise aspirations and satisfy needs; and, on the other hand, to change or cope with the environment. Health is, therefore, seen as a resource for everyday life, not the objective of living; it is a positive concept emphasising social and personal resources, as well as physical capacities.[16]

This is a rich definition, worth considering carefully.

This discussion of 'what is health?' leads on to thinking about what affects people's health.

What Affects Health?

Being healthy is rarely, if ever, the result of chance or luck. A state of health or ill-health, however defined, is the result of a combination of factors having a particular effect on a particular individual at any one time. In order to work towards better health, it is necessary to identify these influential factors. We suggest that you begin by identifying factors which influence your own health, using the following exercise.

Exercise—What affects your health?

The aim of this radiating circle exercise is to identify factors which affect your health. The exercise can be done

- individually
- individually, followed by comparing results with other people
- as a group, pooling your ideas about what influences your health.

You are at the centre of the rings:

In the inner ring, write in factors which influence your health *which are to do with yourself as an individual.*
In the second ring, write in factors which influence your health *which are to do with your immediate social and physical environment.*
In the outer ring, write in factors which influence your health *which are to do with your wider social, physical or political environment.*

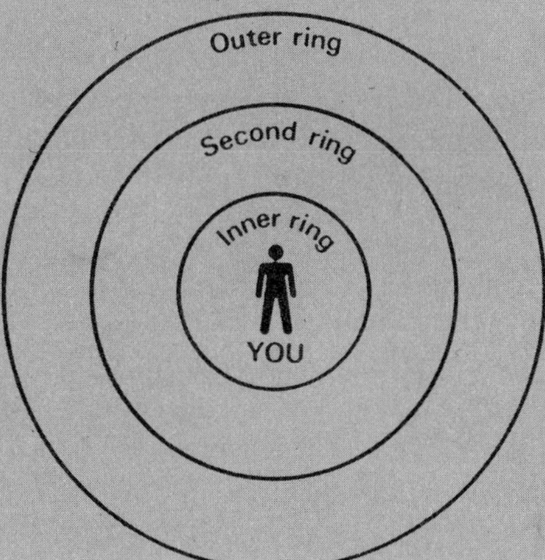

How do these factors influence your health—positively or negatively?
Which factors do you think are the most important?
Are there factors which you have not identified for yourself, but which may be important for other people?[17]

This exercise will have identified a huge range of factors which affect health. They are likely to include genetic make-up, sex, family, religion, culture, friends, income, advertising, social life, social class, race, age, employment status, working conditions, health services, self-esteem, self-confidence, access to leisure facilities and shops, housing, education, national food policy, environmental pollution and many more.

There has been much debate since the early 1970s about the relative importance of these many and varied determinants of health. One of the central concerns has been an increasing awareness that medicine, as a professional practice, has had, surprisingly and disappointingly, little effect on the nation's health. The National Health Service has evolved as a treatment and care service for people who are ill, (a 'National Illness Service'), not as the major means of improving public health.[18] Only about 5 per cent of deaths in the UK today are preventable through good medical treatment. Cancers and heart disease, for example, are the most significant causes of death, but medical care has little impact on the overall death rate from them.[19]

Some people have taken this argument further and claimed that the practice of Western medicine has, in fact, done considerable harm. The side effects of treatment, the complications which set in after surgery, and dependence on prescribed drugs are all examples of this. But more importantly, perhaps, control over health and illness has been taken away from people themselves, who become dependent on doctors and medicines, expecting a cure for every ill and losing their own ability to cope with sickness, disability and death. Aspects of life which may be difficult, such as adolescence, pregnancy and old age, have been increasingly labelled 'medical', and the onus of responsibility shifted from the lay public to the medical profession. These arguments that medicine is, at best, a treatment and care service for the ill and, at worst, a means of undermining people's competence and confidence to improve their health, probably reached a peak around 1980.[20]

Alongside this, a concern has emerged about differences in the health status of different groups of people. This concern grew in the 1970s, with a government working group on inequalities in health leading to the publication of *The Black Report* in 1980. This showed that, for almost every kind of illness and disability, people in the upper socioeconomic classes had a greater chance of avoiding illness and staying healthy than those in the lower classes. It also showed differences in the risks to men compared with those to women, and variations in the apparent 'healthiness' of living in different parts of the country.

All this pointed to the fact that the major determinants of health were concerned with social class, occupation, economic conditions, geographical location and sex. Further evidence towards the end of the 1980s shows that these inequalities are continuing to grow. This means that while *overall* health may have improved, the rate of improvement is not equal across all sections of society. The gap between the health status of the lower social classes compared with the higher social classes continues to become wider. The root cause of these inequalities is social and economic disadvantage which, in turn, is associated with poorer housing, unemployment, stress, poorer nutrition and less social support. Addressing socioeconomic disadvantage is clearly a political issue, and the evidence of increasing inequalities in health shows that it has not yet been satisfactorily addressed.[21]

Case study—Determinants of health

Wendy explains her situation in this way:

'The most influential people in my life are my husband and children. My husband supports me financially and we've got a good secure home—we're buying our house. On the negative side, I feel I'm too dependent on him and I've got no life of my own outside the home. I feel guilty sometimes because I find I actually resent his involvement in his work, even though I know he's working hard for me and the family. The children are lovely, and give me lots of affection. I wouldn't be without them, but I do get fed up with always having to be on tap to meet their demands.

Then there's my mother—even though I only see her once a week she's a strong influence on me. She's always wanting to do things for me—nothing is too much trouble—but this leaves me with the feeling that I'm still a child. I would like to say "no" to her sometimes and not get angry with her. Sometimes I dream about getting a job or even studying for a career, but there are no jobs to be had round here and in any case my husband and mother wouldn't approve of me having a job while the children are still small. I don't feel I can say all this to anyone—they wouldn't understand and it would seem so ungrateful.

I'm overweight and sometimes I find I just stuff myself with sweets and biscuits. It's got worse lately because the mortgage repayments went up and it's very hard to make the housekeeping money go round. So I've not been able to afford much fruit and "healthy" foods; it's cheaper to fill up on chips. I'm worried about money, and recently I haven't been able to sleep properly. I was feeling so depressed that I went to the doctor and he gave me some tablets, but I don't like taking them.

I would like to get out more, but I just can't get myself together.'

Wendy identifies the following positive influences on her health:
- good secure home;
- financial support from her husband;
- affection from her children.

She identifies the following negative influences:
- no jobs available;
- financial worries;
- demanding relationship of children;
- dependent relationship with husband and mother;
- attitude of husband and mother to working outside the home;
- no-one close to her that she can confide in.

The results of these influences are:
- no independent existence outside the home;
- inability to take control, say what she wants and change things;
- negative emotions: guilt, resentment, anger and depression;
- unhealthy behaviours: eating binges, a poor diet, sleeplessness.

continued on next page

continued

These influences, and their consequences for Wendy, reflect the values and attitudes of the society she lives in. They include:

- the expectations for Wendy about a woman's place in society as a carer staying at home, and for Wendy's mother about needing someone to care for;
- the expectation of the role of medicine to solve social and economic problems;
- the expectation that people should bottle up emotions, and women should not assert themselves when it comes to fulfilling their own needs and wants.

In this case study, there is no attempt to look at the root causes of Wendy's ill-health, only to address the difficulties by medication. There is no awareness that education about skills in coping, managing negative emotions, assertiveness, healthy eating on a low budget and group support for losing weight could help Wendy.

Taking a longer-term view, a combination of political change to address job opportunities and rising mortgage rates, education for self-awareness and personal development and a reduction in sexual inequality could prevent many more Wendys ending up in this unhealthy situation.

Addressing the Determinants of Health

So far, we have seen that 'health' is a complex concept, which means different things to different people. We have also seen that the degree of 'healthiness' is linked up with people's ability to reach their full potential. This, in turn, is affected by a wide range of factors which may be broadly classified as lifestyle factors to do with individual health behaviour, and broader social, economic and environmental factors such as social support networks, employment, income and housing.

The focus of health promotion work—whether it is on individual health behaviour or socioeconomic factors—has shifted over the last few decades. Early public health work in the first half of this century concentrated on environmental reforms such as slum clearance, improved sanitation and clean air. Then in the 1950s and 60s the focus shifted towards the need for changes in individual health behaviour about, for example, family planning, venereal disease, accident prevention, immunisation, cervical smear checks, weight control, alcohol consumption and smoking. This emphasis on the 'lifestyle approach' meant a concentration of effort on health education.[22]

During the 1970s, this emphasis became heavily criticised, because it distracted attention from the social and economic determinants of health, and tended to blame individuals for their own ill-health. For example, people with heart disease could be blamed for it because they were overweight and smoked, but the *reasons* for being overweight and smoking were ignored. (Reasons may have included lack of education, no help available to stop smoking, eating and smoking used as a way of coping with stresses such as poor housing or unemployment, lack of availability of cheap nutritious foods, and so on.)[23] This was known as 'victim blaming'.

So in the 1980s, the pendulum swung again and there emerged the broader approach of health promotion which encompassed health education but also addressed the need for political and social action and, importantly, a grass-roots involvement of people themselves in shaping their own health destiny. (There is more about exactly what we mean by the idea of *health promotion* in the next chapter.)

The World Health Organisation has taken a leading role in action for health promotion in the 1980s and 90s. WHO stated in 1977, at the 30th World Health Assembly, that 'The main social target of governments and WHO in the coming decades should be the attainment of all citizens of the world by the year 2000 of a level of health that will permit them to lead a socially and economically productive life'.[24] This was the beginning of what has come to be known as the 'health for all movement' which led to the development of a Regional Strategy for the WHO European Region in 1980.[25]

This regional strategy called for fundamental changes in the health policy of member countries, including a much higher priority for health promotion and disease prevention. It called for not merely the health services but *all* public sectors with a potential impact on health to take positive steps to maintain and improve it. Specific regional targets were set and published in 1985 which emphasised the themes of:

- reducing inequalities in health;
- positive health through health promotion and disease prevention;
- community participation;
- co-operation between health authorities, local authorities and others with an impact on health;
- a focus on primary health care as the main basis of the health care system.

This gave impetus to the new interest in health promotion which we now experience in the 1990s, with its emphasis on addressing inequalities in health through attention to the key social, economic and environmental determinants of ill-health and on community participation in health promotion.

This 'new public health', as it is sometimes known, has found expression in different ways. Examples are:

- the Faculty of Community Medicine published a *Charter for Action* which outlined ways in which the United Kingdom could work towards the achievement of 'health for all by year 2000' in the UK, and produces regular newsletters on progress;[27]
- the Public Health Alliance was formed as an independent voluntary association bringing together individuals and organisations committed to public health;[28]
- WHO set up the 'Healthy Cities' project, which focuses on action for health promotion at city level, aiming to place health high on the agenda of political decision-makers, key groups in the city and the population at large;[29]
- an increasing number of community health projects have been set up, which is a response to the failure of traditional health education to reach the most needy people. They are also a response to the challenge of involving lay people at the grass-roots in identifying the health issues which they set at the top of their agendas, and acting on those issues;[30]
- an upsurge of interest in environmental and ecological health issues as part of the wider 'green' movement.[31]

This chapter has discussed what 'health' is, what affects health, and the ways in which health issues have been addressed over the last few decades. Against this background, we look in the next chapter at what is meant by 'health promotion' and the principles and activities it encompasses.

Notes, References and Further Reading

1 For further reading on concepts of health and illness, see:

Wilson M (1976) *Health is for People*. London: Darton, Longman & Todd
Stott N C H (1983) *Primary Health Care—Bridging the Gap between Theory and Practice*. Berlin/Heidelberg: Springer-Verlag, 33–43
Helman C G (1990) *Culture, Health and Illness*. Guildford, Surrey: Wright
Hart N (1983) *The Sociology of Health and Medicine*. Ormskirk, Lancashire: Causeway Press
Black N, Boswell D, Gray A, Murphey S & Popay J (1984) *Health and Disease: A Reader*. Buckingham: Open University Press, Pt 1

A brief look at international work on the concept of health and concepts of young children is included in Part 2 of:

Kelly P J & Lewis J L (1987) *Education and Health*. Oxford: Pergamon Press

The following book looks at the different philosophies of health in Britain, USA, France and West Germany:

Payer L (1990) *Medicine and Culture*. London: Gollancz

For reading on the concepts of health and illness among ethnic minority groups in Britain, see:

Mares P, Henley A & Baxter C (1985) *Health Care in Multiracial Britain*. Cambridge: National Extension College

For teaching strategies and readings, see:

Mares P, Larbie J & Baxter C (1987) *Trainer's Handbook For Multiracial Health Care*. Cambridge: National Extension College

For a review with particular emphasis on research methodology and theoretical problems of research on concepts of health, see:

Research Unit in Health and Behavioural Change, University of Edinburgh (1989) *Changing the Public Health*. Chichester: Wiley, Ch 3

2 This exercise is adapted, with kind permission from:

The Open University (1980) *The Good Health Guide*. Harmondsworth: Pan Books, p 16 (first published by Harper & Row)

3 The idea for this analysis is based on the findings of an early French study on lay people's concept of health:

Herzlich C (1973) *Health and Illness*. European Monographs in Social Psychology, London: Academic Press

4 Pill R & Stott N (1982) Concepts of illness causation and responsibility; some preliminary data from a sample of working class mothers. *Social Science and Medicine*, **16**, 43–52

5 Blaxter M & Patterson L (1982) *Mothers and Daughters: a Three-generation Study of Health Attitudes and Behaviour*. London: Heinemann Educational Books

6 Williams R (1983) Concepts of health: an analysis of lay logic. *Sociology*, **17**, 185–204

For another study on the health beliefs of older people, see:

Victor C R (1990) What is health? A study of the health beliefs of older people. *Journal of the Institute of Health Education*, **28**(1), 10–15

7 Calnan M (1987) *Health and Illness—The Lay Perspective*. London: Tavistock Publications, Ch 2

8 Calnan M (1987) *Health and Illness—The Lay Perspective*. London: Tavistock Publications

9 On the difficult issue of measuring health status, see:

Hunt S M, McEwan J & McKenna S P (1986) *Measuring Health Status*. London: Croom Helm

Fallowfield L (1990) *The Quality of Life: The Missing Measurement in Health Care*. London: Souvenir Press

Teeling Smith G (1988) *Measuring Health: A Practical Approach*. Chichester: Wiley

10 This issue is dealt with extensively in literature on the sociology of health and illness. For example, see:

Morgan M, Calnan M & Manning N (1985) *Sociological Approaches to Health and Medicine*. London: Croom Helm

Fitzpatrick R, Hinton J, Newnan S, Scambler G & Thompson J (1984) *The Experience of Illness*. London: Tavistock Publications

Richman J (1987) *Medicine and Health*. Harlow: Longman

11 World Health Organisation Constitution 1948

12 World Health Organisation (1984) *Health Promotion: a WHO Discussion Document on the Concepts and Principles*. Reprinted in: *Journal of the Institute of Health Education*, **23**(1), 1985

13 Wilson M (1976) *Health is for People*. London: Darton, Longman & Todd, p 117

14 Seedhouse D (1986) *Health: The Foundations for Achievement*. Chichester: Wiley (Seedhouse writes from a philosopher's point of view)

Aggleton P (1990) *Health*. London: Routledge & Kegan Paul (Aggleton writes as a sociologist)

15 Mansfield K (1977) *Letters and Journals*. London: Pelican Books

Mansfield discusses health in terms of becoming all that she is capable of becoming: this is now a much-quoted phrase.

16 World Health Organisation (1984) *Health Promotion: a WHO Discussion Document on the Concepts and Principles.* Reprinted in: *Journal of the Institute of Health Education*, **23**(1), 1985

17 The 'radiating circle' model is taken from:

Burkitt A (1982) Providing education about health. *Nursing* (June), 29–30. Reproduced by kind permission of Medical Education (International) Ltd

18 For early significant analyses of the determinants of health, including the role of health services, see:

Cochrane A L (1972) *Effectiveness and Efficiency—Random Reflections on Health Services.* Nuffield Provincial Hospitals Trust

McKeown T (1979) *The Role of Medicine: Dream, Mirage or Nemesis.* Oxford: Blackwell

19 Smith A & Jacobson B (eds) (1988) *The Nation's Health: A Strategy for the 1990s.* King Edward's Hospital Fund for London, p 112

20 For further study of this critique of medicine, see:

Illich I (1977) *Limits to Medicine—Medical Nemesis: the Expropriation of Health.* Harmondsworth: Pelican Books

Horrobin D F (1978) *Medical Hubris.* Edinburgh: Churchill Livingstone. Horrobin's book is a reply to Illich's arguments in *Limits to Medicine.*

Inglis B (1981) *Diseases of Civilisation.* London: Hodder & Stoughton

Kennedy I (1981) *The Unmasking of Medicine.* London: Allen & Unwin

21 For review and discussion of inequalities in health, see:

Townsend P, Davidson N & Whitehead M (1988) *Inequalities in Health.* Harmondsworth: Penguin Books. This volume contains *The Black Report* by Townsend & Davidson (first published in 1982) and *The Health Divide* by Whitehead (first published in 1988) together in one volume.

Davey Smith G, Bartley M & Blane D (1990) The Black Report on Socio-economic Inequalities in Health 10 Years On. *British Medical Journal*, **301**, 373–377

Smith A & Jacobson B (eds) (1988) *The Nation's Health: A Strategy for the 1990s.* King Edward's Hospital Fund for London

British Medical Association (1987) *Deprivation and Ill-health.* London: BMA Professional Division

Wilkinson R G (ed) (1986) *Class and Health.* London: Tavistock Publications

Research Unit in Health and Behavioural Change, University of Edinburgh (1989) *Changing the Public Health.* Chichester: Wiley, Ch 6

For a graphic exposition of how family health is affected by the unequal distribution of resources in society, see:

Graham H (1984) *Women, Health and the Family.* Brighton: Wheatsheaf Books/Harvester Press

22 The first major government statement on health education clearly reflects the 'lifestyle approach':

Department of Health and Social Security (1976) *Prevention and Health—Everybody's Business.* London: HMSO

23 For discussion and illustration of the individualistic 'victim-blaming' approach, see:

Rodmell S & Watt A (eds) (1986) *The Politics of Health Education—Raising the Issues*. London: Routledge & Kegan Paul, especially Chs 1 & 2

For research-based argument that classic lifestyle factors (smoking, alcohol, diet and exercise) are important for health, but that social circumstances are more important than lifestyle habits, see:

Blaxter M (1990) *Health and Lifestyles*. London: Tavistock Publications

24 WHO resolution WHO30.43, quoted in:

WHO Regional Office for Europe (1985) *Targets for Health for All*. Copenhagen, Denmark: WHO, p 1

25 WHO Regional Office for Europe (1985) *Targets for Health for All*. Copenhagen, Denmark: WHO

26 For further reading on the 'new public health', see:

Ashton J & Seymour H (1988) *The New Public Health*. Oxford University Press

Martin C & McQueen D (eds) (1989) *Readings for a New Public Health*. Edinburgh University Press

27 Faculty of Community Medicine (1986) *Health For All By The Year 2000: Charter for Action*. London: Faculty of Community Medicine, Royal College of Physicians

Faculty of Public Health Medicine of the Royal College of Physicians. *HFA 2000 News*. Published quarterly. Available from: Faculty of Public Health Medicine, 4 St Andrews Place, Regents Park, London NW1 4LB. Tel: 071 935 0035

28 Public Health Alliance, PO Box 1156, Kings Norton, Birmingham, B30 2AZ

29 Kickbush I (1989) Healthy cities: a working project and a growing movement. *Health Promotion*, **4**(2), 77

Ashton J & Seymour H (1988) *The New Public Health*. Buckingham: Open University Press, Ch 9

30 For reviews of a wide range of community health projects, see:

Community Health Initiatives Resource Unit, National Council for Voluntary Organisations (1987) *Guide to Community Health Projects*. London: CHIRU

Community Projects Foundation, Health Education Authority & Scottish Health Education Group (1988) *Action for Health: Initiatives in Local Communities*. London: Community Projects Foundation, HEA & SHEG

Note: The Community Health Initiatives Resource Unit and The London Community Health Resource combined in 1987 to form The National Community Health Resource, 15 Britannia Street, London WC1 9JP. Among its publications are a newsletter, directories and guides to community health projects, conference reports and books.

For a review of the trend towards community health work, see:

Whitehead M (1989) *Swimming Upstream: Trends and Prospects for Education in Health*. London: King's Fund Institute, 33–36

31 For examples of the 'green' movement linking into health issues, see:

Button J (1989) *How to be Green*. London: Century Hutchinson, 148–170
Grey M & Keeble B (1989) *Greening the NHS*. Letter to *British Medical Journal*, **229** (1 July)

Chapter 2
What is Health Promotion?

Summary

The chapter begins by discussing how to define the term 'health promotion', and outlines the current debate over the difference between the concepts of 'health promotion' and 'health education'. A framework for health promotion activities is proposed, which identifies health promotion as an umbrella term encompassing seven areas of activity. The chapter ends with a brief overview of health promotion competences, indicating where these are discussed in later chapters. Exercises are included to help readers to explore the range of health promotion activities, and the extent of their own health promotion work.

The previous chapter focused on *health*; we now move on to consider the meaning of *health promotion*.

Defining Health Promotion

Health promotion is about raising the health status of individuals and communities. Too often the word *promotion*, when used in the context of health promotion, is associated with sales and advertising, and taken to mean a propaganda approach dominated by the use of the mass media. This is a misunderstanding: by promotion in the health context we mean improving health: advancing, supporting, encouraging and placing it higher on personal and public agendas.

We have seen that major determinants of health are social, economic and environmental, aspects which are often outside individual or even collective control. Therefore, a fundamental aspect of health promotion is that it aims to empower people to have more control over aspects of their lives which affect their health.

These twin elements—improving health and having more control over it—are fundamental to the aims and processes of health promotion. The World Health Organisation's definition of health promotion neatly encompasses this:

> 'Health promotion is the process of enabling people to increase control over, and to improve, their health'.[1]

This definition has become widely adopted.[2]

As discussed in the previous chapter, WHO goes on to say: 'This perspective is derived from a conception of "health" as the extent to which an individual or group is able, on the one hand, to realise aspirations and satisfy needs; and, on the other hand, to change or cope with the environment. Health is, therefore, seen as a resource for everyday life, not the objective of living; it is a positive concept emphasising social and personal resources, as well as physical capacities.'

Health Promotion or Health Education?

There has been much debate since the mid 1980s on the use of the terms *health promotion* and *health education*.[3] The debate came into focus because the range of activities undertaken in the pursuit of better health widened from traditional health education, which was about giving information and working towards individual attitude and behaviour changes.

With rising criticism that this approach was too narrow, focused too much on individual lifestyles and could become 'victim-blaming', more work was done about wider issues. Examples of this are political action to change social policies, putting employee health on the agenda of employers and engaging in community development work for health. This went beyond the scope of traditional health education, and health promotion became widely used as the umbrella term to encompass all these activities. Health education is seen as a very important element in health promotion.

We subscribe to the view that using health promotion as *an umbrella term for a range of activities* is the most useful and practical way forward. However, to avoid misunderstandings and time-consuming arguments about the meaning of words, we need to identify clearly the range of activities which are included in health promotion.[4] This is the subject of the next section.

Before moving to this, though, it is important to appreciate that there is currently no clear, widely adopted consensus of what is meant by 'health promotion'. Some definitions focus on activities, others on aims. The WHO definition we have adopted defines health promotion as a *process* but implies an aim ('enabling people to increase control over, and improve, their health') with a clear philosophical basis of self-empowerment. Perhaps by the end of the century a consensus will have emerged, but for the 1990s, it is necessary to continue to question, research and clarify.[5]

The Scope of Health Promotion

The next exercise aims to start you thinking about the range of activities which may be included in health promotion.

The questions in the exercise give examples of the wide range of activities which may be classified as health promotion. Answering 'yes' to each one indicates a broad view of what may be included: mass media advertising, campaigning on health issues, patient education, self-help, environmental safety measures, public policy issues, health education about physical health, preventive and curative medical procedures,

Exercise—Exploring the scope of health promotion

Consider each of the following statements, and decide whether you think each activity *is* or *is not* health promotion:

	yes	no
1. Using TV advertisements to warn about the dangers of drug use	_____	_____
2. Campaigning for increased taxation of tobacco	_____	_____
3. Explaining to patients how to carry out their doctor's orders	_____	_____
4. Setting up a self-help group for the victims of sexual abuse	_____	_____
5. Providing 'lollipop' people to help children across the road outside schools	_____	_____
6. Raising awareness of how poverty affects health	_____	_____
7. Giving people information about the way their bodies work	_____	_____
8. Immunising children against infectious diseases such as measles	_____	_____
9. Protesting about a breach in the voluntary code of practice for alcohol advertising	_____	_____
10. Running low-cost, keep fit classes for older people at local leisure centres	_____	_____
11. Providing 'healthier' menu choices at workplace canteens	_____	_____
12. Teaching a programme of personal and social education in a secondary school	_____	_____
13. Providing support to mentally handicapped people living in the community	_____	_____

What were your reasons for saying 'yes' or 'no'? Can you identify the criteria you are using for deciding whether an activity is 'health promotion'?

codes of practice on health issues, health-enhancing facilities in local communities, workplace health policies and social education for young people. Answering 'no' indicates that you identify criteria which exclude these activities from the realms of 'health promotion'. For example, you may have said 'no' to Question 2 because increasing tobacco taxation would place a heavier burden on smokers in poor financial circumstances thus putting their health even more at risk.

The many attempts to provide frameworks for classifying health promotion activities have helped to clarify the issues.[5] Drawing on these, we propose to start by focusing on *identifying the activities* which contribute to better health (Fig. 1). This is a pragmatic approach to a complex issue, which we adopt because this book is a practical guide to health promotion, and it will provide a framework for identifying the competences health promoters used. (We clarify what we mean by 'competences' later in this chapter.) Figure 1 maps out all those activities which aim to improve people's health. The first point to note is that there are two sets of activities: those which are

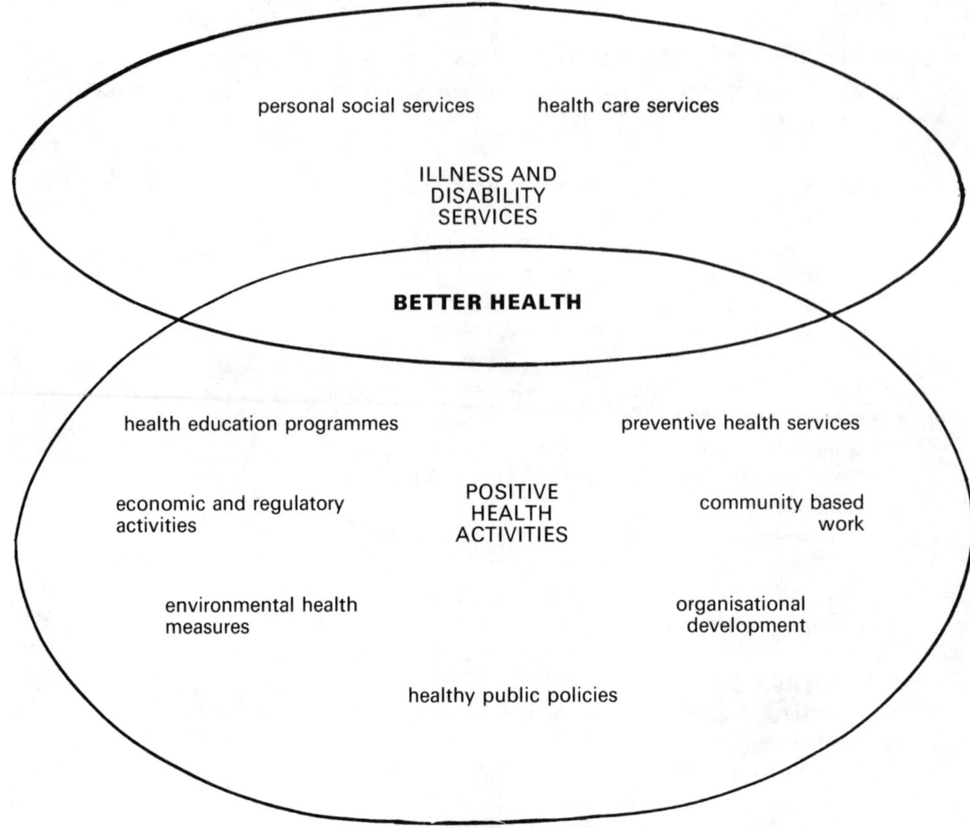

Fig. 1 Activities for better health.

about providing services for the ill and disabled, and positive health activities which are about personal, social and environmental changes aiming to prevent ill-health and develop healthier living conditions and ways of life. These two sets of activities overlap, because they both contribute to better health, and they are often closely related in practice. We identify nine categories of activities, comprised of two illness and disability services and seven types of positive health activities, as follows:

Illness and Disability Services

Personal social services. This category includes all those social services which aim to address the needs of sick or disabled members of society whose health (in its widest sense) is improved by those services. It includes, for example, community care of the elderly and home help services.

Health care services. This includes the major work of the health services: treatment, cure and care in primary care and hospital settings.

We now need to address a difficult issue: if all illness and disability services promote better health, which they obviously do, are they all called 'health promotion'? For example, is taking out someone's appendix, or placing a child in a foster home, health promotion? This is not just a quibble about words. It is an important question when considering the boundaries of service provision by health promotion agencies, of the many courses designed to educate health promoters in the necessary skills and knowledge, and, indeed, of this book.

It is helpful to go back to our definition of health promotion, 'enabling people to increase control over, and improve, their health'. Things which need to be done *to* people (like taking out their appendix or placing them in a foster home) are excluded from this definition, so these are generally *not* considered to be health promotion activities. But those aspects of care and treatment which *are* about enabling people to take control over their health and improve it, such as educating patients in the skills of self-care, or educating foster parents in the skills of parenting, *are* legitimate areas of health promotion. So is creating a health-promoting environment by, for example, modifying a home to make it suitable for a disabled person.

Positive Health Activities:

Health education programmes are planned opportunities for people to learn about health, and to undertake voluntary changes in their behaviour. Such programmes may include providing information, exploring values and attitudes, making health decisions and acquiring skills to enable behaviour change to take place. They involve promoting self-esteem and self-empowerment so that people are enabled to take action about their health. They can happen on a personal one-to-one level such as health visitor/client, teacher/pupil, in a group such as a smoking cessation group or exercise class, or by means of reaching large audiences through the mass media, health fairs or exhibitions.

As we have already discussed, health education programmes may also be a part of health care and personal social services, and because of this it is useful to understand the concept of *primary, secondary* and *tertiary health education.*

Primary health education is directed at healthy people, and aims to prevent ill-health arising in the first place. Most health education for children and young people falls into this category, dealing with such topics as hygiene, contraception, nutrition and social skills and personal relationships, and aiming to build up a positive sense of self-worth in children. Primary health education is concerned not merely with helping to prevent illness, but with positively improving the quality of health and thus the quality of life.

There is also often a major role for health education when people are ill. It may be possible to prevent ill-health moving to a chronic or irreversible stage, and to restore people to their former state of health. This is known as *secondary* health education —educating patients about their condition and what to do about it. Restoring good health may involve the patient in changing behaviour (such as stopping smoking) or in complying with a therapeutic regime and, possibly, learning about self-care and self-help. Clearly, health education of the patient is of great importance if treatment and therapy are to be effective and illness is not to recur.

But there are, of course, many patients whose ill-health has not been, or could not be, prevented and who cannot be completely cured. There are also people with permanent disabilities and handicaps. *Tertiary* health education is concerned with educating patients and their relatives about how to make the most of the remaining potential for healthy living, and how to avoid unnecessary hardship, restrictions and complications. Rehabilitation programmes contain a considerable amount of tertiary health education.

However, it is not always easy to see where people fit into this primary, secondary or tertiary framework because, as we have already seen, a person's state of health is open to interpretation. For example, is educating an overweight person who appears to be perfectly well despite their weight primary or secondary health education?

Examples—Primary, secondary and tertiary health education

	Nutrition	*Road Accidents*
Primary health education	Education about adequate and balanced food providing enough nutrients, fibre and energy.	Accident prevention, including campaigning for safer roads and vehicles, as well as educating individuals about safe practices.
Secondary health education	How to adjust eating habits in cases of overweight or other reversible health problems, such as maturity-onset diabetes.	How to give first aid after an accident to maximise chances of full recovery.
Tertiary health education	How to adjust eating habits to ensure maximum health and minimum complications in chronic incurable conditions, such as juvenile-onset diabetes or food allergies.	Rehabilitation training to maximise potential for healthy living following accident causing permanent disability, such as loss of a limb or paralysis.

Preventive health services. These include medical services which aim to prevent ill-health, such as immunisation, family planning and personal health checks, as well as wider preventive health services such as child protection services for children at risk of abuse.

Community-based work. This is a 'bottom-up' approach to health promotion, working with and for people, involving communities in health work such as local campaigns for better facilities. It includes community development, which is essentially about communities identifying their own health needs and taking action to address them. The sort of activities which may result could include forming self-help and pressure groups, and developing local health-enhancing facilities and services.

Organisational development. This is about developing and implementing policies within organisations which promote the health of staff and customers. Examples include implementing policies on equal opportunities, providing healthy food choices in staff dining rooms and working with commercial organisations to develop and promote 'healthier' products, such as leaner meat, lower-fat spreads and cheeses, low and non-alcoholic drinks and biodegradable packaging.

Healthy public policies. Developing and implementing healthy public policies is what the 'new public health' is about.[6] It involves statutory and voluntary agencies, professionals and the public working together to develop changes in the conditions of living. It is about seeing the implications for health in policies about, for example, equal opportunities, housing, employment, transport and leisure. Good public transport, for example, would improve health by reducing the number of cars on the road, lessening pollution, using less fuel and reducing the stress of the daily grind of travelling for commuters. It could also reduce isolation for those who do not own cars and enable people to have access to shopping and leisure facilities—all measures which improve well-being.

Environmental health measures. This is about making the physical environment conducive to health, whether at home, at work or in public places. It includes traditional public health measures such as providing clean food and water and controlling pollution, as well as working on newer issues such as smoke-free areas in restaurants and pubs, and controlling the use of environmentally damaging chlorofluorocarbons (CFCs).

Economic and regulatory activities. This is political and educational activity directed at politicians, policy-makers and planners, involving lobbying for and implementing legislative changes such as food labelling regulations, pressing for voluntary codes of practice such as those which relate to alcohol advertising, or advocating financial measures such as increases in tobacco taxation.

A Framework for Health Promotion Activities

Having identified the health education aspects of personal social services and health care services as health promotion, and identified seven areas of positive health activity, we propose the following framework (Figure 2). There are two important points to make about the use of this framework. The first is that activities do not always fall tidily into categories. For example, would a health visitor who was supporting a local women's health group be engaged in *a health education programme* because she provided health information to the group and set up stress management sessions, or *community-based work* because some members of the group had got together to lobby their local health services for better family planning facilities? Would an environmental health officer concerned about air pollution levels on a factory site be engaged in *organisational development* because she was working towards healthier working conditions for the staff, or *environmental health measures* because she aimed to achieve cleaner air for the local community?

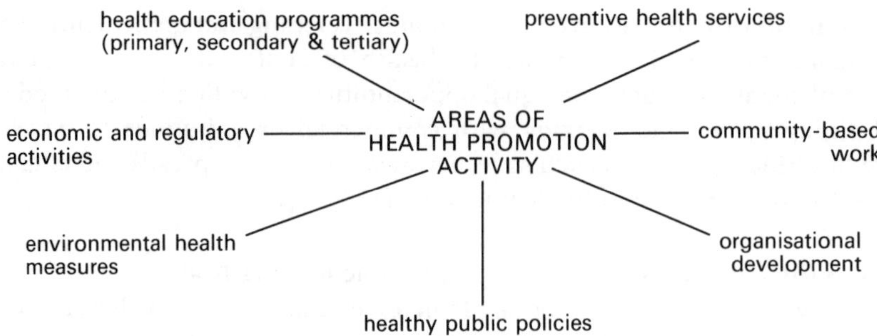

Fig. 2 A framework for health promotion activities.

Obviously, areas of activity do overlap but this is not important. What *is* important is to appreciate the range of activities encompassed by health promotion, and the many ways in which you can contribute to improvements in health status.

The second point about using this framework is to note that we are talking about planned, deliberate activities, and it is important to recognise that a great deal of health promotion happens informally and incidentally. For example, portrayal of damage caused by excessive drinking in a television soap opera, provision of low-cost exercise classes by a local entrepreneur and an advertising campaign to promote wholewheat breakfast cereals, are all health promotion activities which are not likely to be planned with specific health promotion aims in mind. They may, however, be significant influences for change.

The next exercise is designed to help you to identify your own contribution to health promotion.

Exercise—Identifying your health promotion work

Look at the following diagram (it is the same as Figure 2) which identifies seven major areas of health promotion activity. On a sheet of paper, list the seven headings, and note down against each one any parts of your work which you think come into that category (if you are not sure what each category includes, look back at the explanations).

Then think about each category again, and consider whether there is scope for developing your work within each category.

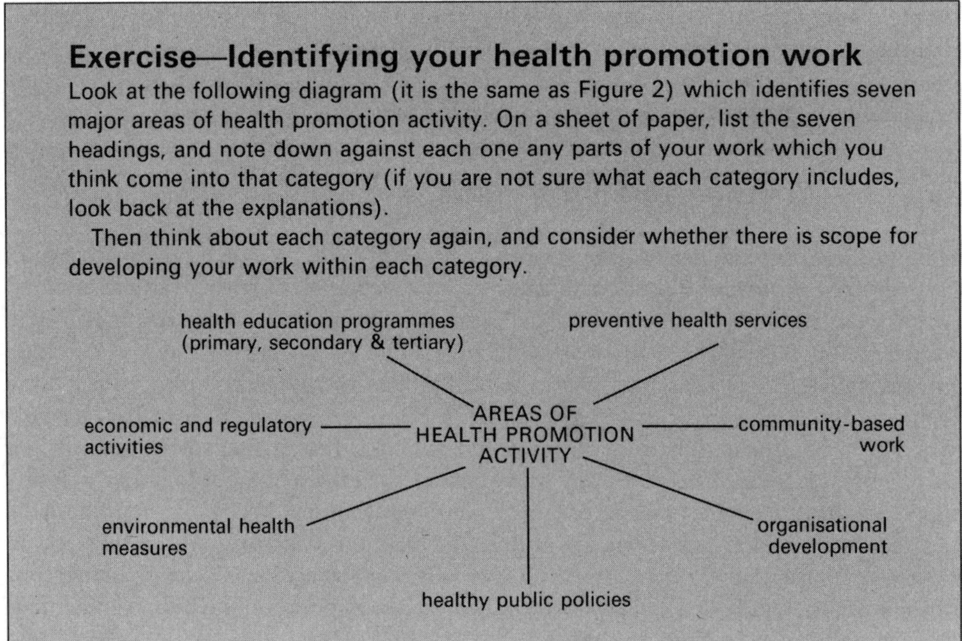

Developing Competence in Health Promotion

Having mapped out the *activities* the health promoter may be engaged in, we now look at the *skills and methods* used when those activities take place; in other words, we are considering the *competences* which health promoters need to develop. By 'competences' we mean the specific combination of knowledge, attitudes and skills needed to do a particular job.

It is useful to think that there are, broadly, two aspects of your work to consider. One is the *technical/specialist aspect*: immunising a child, taking a cervical smear, recording blood pressure, undertaking microbiological tests for food hygiene purposes, enforcing legislation, building safer roads, interpreting welfare rights legislation or damp-proofing a home. All of these are the subject of specialist training, and outside the scope of this book.

The other aspect of your work is about *working with people* to promote health in many different situations with a variety of different aims. To do this, you need to have knowledge of particular methods and acquire special skills. We do not claim that these are exclusive to health promotion work, but they are the core competences of health promotion. We identify them as follows.

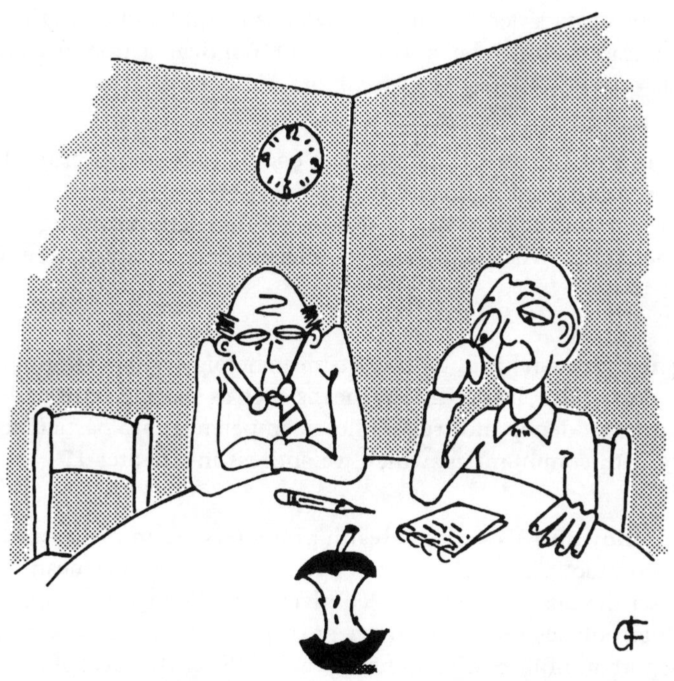

Acquiring core competence in health promotion

Core Competences in Health Promotion

Managing, Planning and Evaluating. Managing resources for health promotion, including money, materials, oneself and other people, are crucial. Systematic planning is needed for effective and efficient health promotion. All health promotion work also requires evaluation, and different methods are appropriate for different approaches. All these are addressed in Part 2 *Moving from Theory to Practice*, Chapters five, six and seven.

Communicating. Health promotion is about people, so competence in communication is essential and fundamental. A high level of competence is needed in one-to-one communication and in working with groups in various ways, both formal and informal. Communication is addressed in Chapters eight, nine and ten.

Educating. Educating about health requires good communication, but it also requires additional educational competence so that health educators can work in different settings such as formal lecturing or informal group work, and select and use appropriate strategies for different educational goals.

Educational competence is obviously used in health education programmes, but it is also used when undertaking other kinds of activities. For example, patient education is an integral part of preventive health services, education on policy implementation (such as a healthy food policy) is part of organisational development, public education is part of implementing an environmental health measure and educating members of statutory organisations may be a key part of political action for social change. Education is addressed in Chapters 11, 14 and 15.

Marketing and Publicising. This requires competence in, for example, marketing and advertising, using local radio and getting local press coverage of health issues. It may be used when undertaking any health promotion activities which would benefit from wider publicity. Marketing and publicising are addressed in Chapters 14 and 15.

Facilitating and Networking. By this we mean helping others to promote their own and other people's health, using various means such as sharing skills and information, and building up confidence and trust. These competences are particularly important when working with communities, which we address in Chapter 12.

Influencing Policy and Practice. Health promoters are in the business of influencing policies and practices which affect health. (By 'policies' we mean broad plans of action, which set the direction for detailed planning.) These can be at any level, from national (such as policies set by government or political parties, about, for example, housing, transport and future directions for the NHS) to the level of day-to-day work of a health promoter (such as what sort of health promotion clinics will be run in a GP practice, or what resources will be devoted to specific health promotion activities in an environmental health department).

In order to influence policy and practice, you need to understand how power is distributed and exercised between people at any level, from a group of colleagues to those in positions of great authority or influence, and to be able to use that knowledge to affect decisions. This includes working with statutory, voluntary and commercial

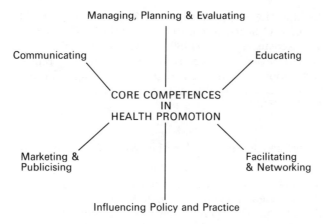

Fig. 3 Core competences in health promotion.

organisations to influence them to develop health promoting policies for their staff and to produce health-enhancing products and services. It also includes working for healthy public policies and economic and regulatory changes requiring lobbying and taking political action. These competences are addressed in Chapter 13.

These six clusters of competences are not exhaustive. As health promotion work grows and develops, and as it is practised in a variety of innovatory ways, there will be many more methods adopted and skills required. This is to be welcomed; what we aim to do here is to identify current core competences and help you to acquire these.

It is clearly unrealistic to expect all health promoters to be highly competent in all aspects of health promotion. A practice nurse, for example, will work predominantly in health education and preventive health services, needing a high level of competence in communication and education. However, she also needs other competences in order to plan and evaluate her work, market her health promotion programmes to her patients, facilitate change in her patients and be able to refer them to a network of helpful contacts. She will also need to be able to influence the development of health promotion policy in her practice.

All the six areas of competence we have identified are fundamental to health promotion activities, but you will probably find that you need some to a greater degree than others. They will be acquired in a variety of ways, including your life experience outside work, basic training, in-service training and work experience.

Notes, References and Further Reading

1 World Health Organisation (1984) *Health Promotion: a WHO Discussion Document on the Concepts and Principles.* Reprinted in: *Journal of the Institute of Health Education*, **23**(1), 1985

2 See, for example:

Whitehead M (1989) *Swimming Upstream: Trends and Prospects in Education for Health.* London: King's Fund Institute, p 7

The Health Education Authority and the Society of Health Education & Health Promotion Officers, in consultation with the Department of Health, produced a consensus report in 1989 on the role of health education/promotion departments within the NHS. In it, they state that 'The purpose of a health education/promotion department is regarded as being: "To promote the health of the local population by enabling people to increase control over and improve their health."' (HEA 1989)

3 A series of short articles appeared in the *Health Education Journal* in 1984/5:

Seymour H (1984) Health education versus health promotion—a practitioner's view. *Health Education Journal*, **43**(2 & 3), 87–88
Catford J & Nutbeam D (1984) Towards a definition of health education and health promotion. *Health Education Journal*, **43**(2 & 3), 38
Speller V (1985) Defining health promotion: service implications. *Health Education Journal*, **44**(2), 96
French J (1985) To educate or promote health? *Health Education Journal*, **44**(3), 115–116
Tannahill A (1985) What is health promotion? *Health Education Journal*, **44**(4), 167–168

4 For a useful glossary of health promotion terms, including health education, health promotion, disease prevention, community development, positive health, health policy, health status, life skills, new public health, self-empowerment, and many more, see:

Nutbeam D (1986) Health promotion glossary. *Health Promotion*, **1**(1), 119–127

5 In this chapter, we draw particularly on:

Catford J & Nutbeam D (1984) Towards a definition of health education and health promotion. *Health Education Journal*, **43**(2 & 3), 38
Nutbeam D & Catford J C (1986) Health promotion in action: practical ideas for programme implementation. *Health Promotion*, **1**(2) 187–90

See also:

Anderson R (1984) Health promotion: an overview. In *European Monographs in Health Education Research, No. 6* (ed Baric, L) Edinburgh: Scottish Health Education Group
World Health Organisation (1984) *Health Promotion: a WHO Discussion Document on the Concepts and Principles*. Reprinted in: *Journal of the Institute of Health Education*, **23**(1) 1985
Tannahill A (1985) What is health promotion? *Health Education Journal*, **44**(4), 167–168
Downie R S, Fyfe C & Tannahill A (1990) *Health Promotion: Models and Values*. Oxford: Oxford University Press, Pt 1
Tones K, Tilford S & Robinson Y (1990) *Health Education: Effectiveness and Efficiency*. London: Chapman & Hall, Ch 1

French J (1990) Boundaries and horizons, the role of health education within health promotion. *Health Education Journal*, **49**(1), 7–10

6 Ashton J & Seymour H (1988) *The New Public Health.* Buckingham: Open University Press, Ch 6

Chapter 3
Philosophical Issues in Health Promotion

Summary

This chapter identifies and explores some key philosophical issues inherent in health promotion practice. Two fundamental questions about the aims of health promotion are explored: to change the individual or change society, and, to ensure compliance with a health promotion programme or to enable clients to make an informed choice? A framework of five approaches to health promotion provides the reader with a tool for analysing key aims and values. Two exercises and a case study are included. The chapter goes on to discuss eight more ethical issues, and a framework of questions to help health promoters to make ethical decisions. A suggested code of practice and two more exercises complete the chapter.

In this chapter, we tease out some of the key philosophical issues in health promotion. We encourage you to think deeply about *why* you are engaging in specific activities, what values are reflected in your work and what ethical dilemmas are presented. We consider guidelines on how to approach ethical decision-making and some key principles of practice.

Philosophical issues are important.[1] Health promotion work, if successful, will affect the lives of other people and it would be irresponsible to equip you with practical skills without also helping you to understand the values and ethics implicit in your work.

First, we look at the aims of health promotion.

Clarifying Health Promotion Aims

Aiming to Change the Individual or Change Society?

Throughout the last decade there has been much debate over different approaches (often called models) of health education and health promotion.[2] (See Chapter Two.) Much of the debate centres around the *aims* of the work. A key question is: should it aim to change individual behaviour and lifestyles, or to change the socioeconomic and physical environment?

As we discussed in Chapter One, a great deal of traditional health education has aimed to change the behaviour of individuals towards healthier lifestyles. In other words, it aims to change people to fit the environment, and has done little to make the environment a healthier place to live in. It has also resulted in 'blaming the victims' for their own ill-health, which is an ethical issue health educators need to face. On the other hand, it can be argued that individuals often *can* do something to improve their own health, that they want to take responsibility for themselves and that health education is an essential tool in that process. It is also argued that sensitive health education can promote people's self-esteem and confidence, empowering them to take more control over their own health.

Proponents of the lifestyle change approach also argue that medical and health experts have the knowledge which enables them to know what is in the best interests of their patients and the public at large, and that it is their responsibility to persuade people to adopt the 'healthiest' measures. Furthermore, society has vested that responsibility with them, and people often seek advice and help in health matters; it is not necessarily a matter of persuading clients against their will. Sometimes, too, individuals may not be in a position to take responsibility for themselves because they may be too young, too ill, or mentally handicapped.

There are several points to be taken into account if the lifestyle change aim is pursued. Firstly, you cannot assume that lay people believe that 'experts' know best. The public perceives experts to constantly change their minds, over, for example, whether jogging does more harm than good, whether there really is a danger that HIV infection will be spread by heterosexual contact or whether living near a nuclear power plant is hazardous to health. Sometimes the 'experts' are proved wrong.

Secondly, there is a danger of imposing alien values on a client. Frequently, this is the imposition of white, middle-class values on working-class people. For example, a doctor may perceive that the most important thing for a patient is losing weight and lowering blood pressure, but drinking beer in the pub with friends may be far more important to the overweight, middle-aged, unemployed patient. Who is to say which set of values is 'right'? Whose life is it anyway?

Thirdly, pushing a lifestyle change approach may produce negative and counterproductive feelings: of guilt for failing to comply, or rebelliousness and anger at being told what to do.

Fourthly, we cannot assume that individual behaviour is the primary cause of ill health. This a limited view, as we have seen when looking at determinants of health and inequalities in health in Chapter One. There is a danger that focusing on the individual distracts attention from the more significant (and, of course, politically sensitive) determinants of health such as the socioeconomic conditions of racism, poverty, housing and unemployment.

Finally, we also cannot assume that individuals have a genuine freedom to choose 'health' lifestyles. Freedom to choose is often very limited. Economic factors may affect the choice of food because, for example, fresh fruit and wholemeal bread are relatively more expensive than biscuits and white bread. Social factors are also important: there is very little real freedom of choice about smoking for adolescents whose parents and friends all smoke, and who risk ridicule if they do not. Also, how much freedom do people really have to change other health-demoting factors such as stressful working conditions and unemployment? It is easy to become 'victim-blaming': blaming people for their own ill-health when in fact they are the victims of their circumstances. In situations where resources of time, energy and income are limited, health choices become health compromises. What a health promoter may see as irresponsibility may actually be what the client sees as the most responsible action in the circumstances.[3]

It is crucially important that everyone engaged in health promotion should be aware of these ethical issues and have an opportunity to consider them in relation to their own work, particularly if they are engaged in health education with the aim of changing individual lifestyles. The following exercise is designed to help you to think through the issues.

Exercise—Analysing your philosophy of health promotion[4]

Consider the following statements A and B:

A. The key aim of health promotion is to inform people about the ways in which their behaviour and lifestyle can affect their health, to ensure that the information is understood, to help them explore their values and attitudes, and (where appropriate) to help them to change their behaviour.

B. The key aim of health promotion is to raise awareness of the many socioeconomic policies at national and local level (eg. employment, housing, food subsidies, advertising, transport and health service policies) which are not conducive to good health, and to actively work towards a change in those policies.

1. Taking Statement A:
   —list arguments in support of this view;
   —list any points about the limitations of this view, and any arguments against it.
2. Do the same with Statement B.
3. Do you think that the views in A and B are *complementary* or *incompatible*? Why?
4. Imagine these two views at either end of a spectrum:

   A |. . . . . |. . . . . |. . . . . |. . . . . |. . . . . | B
   1 2 3 4 5

   Indicate the two positions on the scale of 1 to 5 which most closely reflect (a) *what you actually do* in practice and (b) *what you would like to do* if you were free to work exactly as you would wish to.

Part Three of this book *Developing Competence in Health Promotion* addresses how you can promote health in a way which is sensitive to these issues, and Chapter 13 *Changing Policy and Practice* looks particularly at what you can do to challenge and change health-related policies.

Aiming for Compliance or Informed Choice?

Another key question about the aims of health promotion centres on what you aim to do with or for the client (whether the client is a single individual, a community, or an organisation). Is your aim to ensure that your client complies with your programme, using a mixture of education, publicity and persuasion as required? Or is it to enable your client to make an informed choice, and have the skills and confidence to carry that choice through into action, whatever that choice may be?

To take an example: suppose a health promoter is working with a client whose sexual behaviour is such that there is a serious risk of catching sexually transmitted diseases, and even HIV. If the aim is *compliance* it is more likely that the health promoter will be persuasive, will stress the risks to the client, and will consider the session a failure if the client does not choose to behave differently. If, on the other hand, the health promoter's aim is to enable the client to make an informed choice, the health promoter will ensure that the client understands the facts and the risks, will put a lot of effort into encouraging and supporting the client and accept that if the client chooses *not* to change behaviour, this choice will be respected. It would not be interpreted as a failure, because the client made an informed choice.

The same issues arise with health promotion work on a larger scale. Is the aim of a campaign to ban a nuclear power station, for example, to persuade people to a particular point of view or to give them the information on which to make up their own minds?

This is a difficult question. Most health promoters are doing their jobs because they believe that the action they are advocating is in the best interests of individuals and society as a whole. It raises questions about how far to go in imposing your own values and ideas of what is 'good' and 'right' on other people.

Analysing Your Aims and Values: Five Approaches

In our view, there is no one 'right' aim for health promotion, and no one 'right' approach or set of activities. We need to work out for ourselves which aim and which activities we use, in accordance with our own professional code of conduct (if there is one), our own carefully considered values and our own assessment of our clients needs.

Different models of health promotion and health education are a useful *tool of analysis,* which can help you to clarify your own aims and values. We identify a framework of five approaches to health promotion, and suggest some of the values implicit in any particular approach.

The medical approach: the aim of this approach is freedom from medically-defined disease and disability, such as infectious diseases, cancer and heart disease. The approach involves medical intervention to prevent or ameliorate ill-health, possibly using a persuasive or paternalistic method—for example, persuading parents to bring their children for immunisation, women to use family planning clinics and middle-aged men to be screened for high blood pressure. This approach values preventive medical procedures, and the medical profession's responsibility to ensure that patients comply with recommended procedures.

The behaviour change approach: the aim of this approach is to change people's individual attitude and behaviour, so that they adopt a 'healthy' lifestyle (as defined by you or your employing organisation). Examples include teaching people how to stop smoking, education about 'sensible' drinking, encouraging people to take more exercise, look after their teeth, eat the 'right' foods, and so on. Those using this approach will be convinced that a 'healthy' lifestyle is in the best interests of the clients, and will see it as their responsibility to encourage as many people as possible to adopt the 'healthy' lifestyle they advocate.

The educational approach: the aim of this approach is to give information and ensure knowledge and understanding of health issues, and to enable well-informed decisions to be made. Information about health is presented, and people are helped to explore their values and attitudes, and make their own decisions. Help in carrying out those decisions and adopting new health practices may also be offered. School health education programmes, for example, emphasise helping pupils to learn the skills of healthy living, not merely to acquire the knowledge. Those favouring this approach will value the educational process, will respect the right of individuals to choose their own health behaviour, and will see it as their responsibility to raise with them the health issues which they think will be in their clients' best interests.

The client-centred approach: the aim of this approach is to work with clients in order to help them to identify what they want to know about and take action on, and make their own decisions and choices according to their own interests and values. The health promoter's role is to act as a facilitator, helping people to identify their concerns and gain the knowledge and skills they require to make changes happen. Self-empowerment of the client is seen as central to this aim.[5] Clients are valued as equals who have knowledge, skills and abilities to contribute, and who have an absolute right to control their own health destinies.

The societal change approach: the aim of this approach is to effect changes on the physical, social and economic environment, in order to make it more conducive to good health. The focus is on changing society, not on changing the behaviour of individuals. Those using this approach will value their democratic right to change society, will be committed to putting health on the political agenda at all levels and to the importance of shaping the health environment rather than shaping the individual lives of the people who live in it.

FIVE APPROACHES TO HEALTH PROMOTION SUMMARY AND EXAMPLE

	AIM	HEALTH PROMOTION ACTIVITY	IMPORTANT VALUES	EXAMPLE—SMOKING
MEDICAL	Freedom from medically-defined disease and disability	Promotion of medical intervention to prevent or ameliorate ill-health	Patient compliance with preventive medical procedures	*Aim*—freedom from lung disease, heart disease and other smoking-related disorders *Activity*—encourage people to seek early detection and treatment of smoking related disorders
BEHAVIOUR CHANGE	Individual behaviour conducive to freedom from disease	Attitude and behaviour change to encourage adoption of 'healthier' lifestyle	Healthy life style as defined by health promoter	*Aim*—behaviour changes from smoking to not smoking *Activity*—persuasive education to prevent non-smokers from starting and persuade smokers to stop
EDUCATIONAL	Individuals with knowledge and understanding enabling well informed decisions to be made and acted upon	Information about cause and effects of health-demoting factors. Exploration of values and attitudes. Development of skills required for healthy living	Individual right of free choice. Health promoter's responsibility to identify educational content	*Aim*—clients will have understanding of the effects of smoking on health. They will make a decision whether to smoke or not and act on this decision *Activity*—giving information to clients about the effects of smoking. Helping them to explore their own values and attitudes and come to a decision. Helping them to learn how to stop smoking if they want to
CLIENT CENTRED	Working with clients on the clients' own terms	Working with health issues, choices and actions which clients identify. Empowering the client	Clients as equals. Clients' right to set agenda. Self-empowerment of client	Anti-smoking issue is only considered if clients identify it as a concern. Clients identify what, if anything, they want to know and do about it
SOCIETAL CHANGE	Physical and social environment which enables choice of healthier lifestyle	Political/social action to change physical/ social environment	Right and need to make environment health-enhancing	*Aim*—make smoking socially unacceptable, so it is easier not to smoke than to smoke *Activity*—no smoking policy in all public places. Cigarette sales less accessible, especially to children, promotion of non-smoking as social norm. Limiting and challenging tobacco advertising and sports sponsorship

Exercise—Identifying your aims and values

Select two or three specific health promotion activities you are engaged in, such as a group health education programme, a publicity campaign, a patient-education scheme, an immunisation programme, a one-to-one meeting with a client, a community activity or working on a health policy. Select different kinds of activities if you can.

With reference to the chart 'Five approaches to health promotion', identify which approach you are using for each activity (you may find that you will identify more than one approach).

For each activity, define the aim and the important values implicit in your work (you may find it helpful to look at the 'Case studies—approaches in practice').

Discuss your findings with a partner or in a small group.

Case studies—approaches in practice

Jill is a hospital nurse running a programme of rehabilitation for patients who have had heart attacks. She decides that she is working with an educational approach, aiming for her patients to make informed decisions and have knowledge and skills about taking exercise, modifying their diet, etc. She accepts that some patients will choose not to do so. She thinks that sometimes she may be working in a behavioural change model, because she sincerely believes that her patients would be better off if they changed their behaviour and she finds that she really wants to persuade them sometimes. In the end, she decides that it is their choice and their life, and that she will not pressure them into doing what they do not want to do. Jill is aware, though, that some of her colleagues (who favour the behavioural change approach) think she should be tougher and shock the patients into complying by horror stories of what may happen to them if they do not.

Terry is a community worker, based in a deprived housing estate. Facilities for recreation, exercise and buying good food (among other things) are poor. He decides that he is working with a mixture of client-centred and societal-change approaches, because people in the community have identified that they want a better diet, and he is helping them to set up a food co-operative and help each other to learn new cooking skills. He is also helping them to lobby their local councillor for better green spaces on the estate where the children can play.

Some More Ethical Dilemmas

Bottom-up or Top-down?

There is a key issue of control and power at the heart of health promotion work. Who decides what work will be done: who sets the agenda? Is it 'bottom-up', set by people themselves identifying issues they perceive as relevant, or is it 'top-down', set by health promoters who have the power and resources to make decisions and impose their own ideas of what should be done?

Put this way, it appears to be a straightforward polarised choice; in practice, of course, it is not so simple. The issue can be considered at different levels. For example, at the level of an individual health promoter there is a spectrum of possible positions which could be taken: at one end, coercion or persuasion, then giving advice, then a more neutral position of giving the facts but leaving the client to decide, to the position at the other end of the spectrum: the health promoter who listens, gives information when asked but never offers advice or even an opinion.

At national level, certain health promotion priorities are identified by government with the advice of professionals. These programmes are then imposed on the population who may or may not perceive them as relevant. But ultimately the decision to implement these programmes is that of the government elected by the people, so we come full circle.

There is also a danger that when the public is involved in health promotion at a local level, local people can be manipulated into changing their agenda to match that of the health promoters. Community development should be about empowering the public to work on their own agendas of health issues, even if these are radically different from the agendas of those working for health in a professional capacity. But health promoters have a responsibility to raise awareness of health issues, provide information about them and create demand for change, so where does this process differ from manipulating the community into wanting what the health promoters desired in the first place?

Perhaps one way forward is to be aware of the necessity to be absolutely honest and open about your aims and the limitations of your freedom to act on other people's agenda issues.

Just Widening the Inequalities?

As discussed in Chapter One, there are wide differences in the health status of different groups of people, and generally those in poorer social and economic conditions are the least healthy, with the gap between the health status of rich and poor becoming ever wider.

There is a danger that health promotion activities only reach the better-off, who have the time, money and education to make use of health information and take health action. Those who are trapped in poor financial circumstances and who struggle to survive are less likely to be in a position to change their lifestyle or devote their energies to lobbying for social or political changes. There is clearly a need to be sensitive to this, and to ensure that health promotion is relevant to those most in need.

The Health Promoter: a Shining Example?

Consider the cases of an overweight dietitian, a nurse who smokes and an environmental health officer who does not use unleaded petrol. All three are in a position where they need to address these issues as part of their work and possibly be asked for advice which they clearly do not follow themselves.

Few health promoters would claim that they are perfect examples of healthy living, but we suggest that they have a responsibility to consider their own health, ways in which it could be improved, and ways in which they could contribute to a healthier environment. Health promoters are teaching by example, and the examples discussed above convey silent messages that it is OK to be overweight, to smoke or to pollute the atmosphere with leaded petrol. It is probably best to be open and honest in situations where health promoters' own lifestyles are at odds with the health-promoting ways they are advocating. Personal experience can also be turned to good advantage: for example, if the dietitian has a constant struggle to control her own weight, she can use that experience to develop a greater understanding of her clients' difficulties.

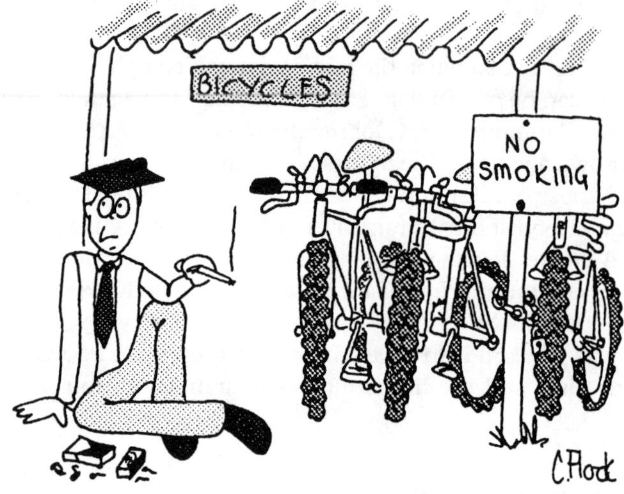

Few health promoters would claim that they are perfect examples of healthy living

Facts, Fads or Fashions?

A common complaint from the public is that experts keep changing their minds, and there are many examples which illustrate this, such as constantly changing information about environmental hazards and how to reduce them or controversy about the value of cholesterol testing. Health issues go in and out of the news, and come to be seen as fads or fashions with little solid foundation in fact and, certainly, low credibility.

A difficulty is that research continuously turns up new information, often controversial and not accepted as generally 'received wisdom' until it has been independently confirmed from new sources: this may take many years. But media attention focuses on the new and controversial, so the public becomes alerted to the debates.

At what point do you decide that the evidence is sufficiently convincing to begin publicising a new message, or to campaign to change an aspect of healthy policy or legislation? If you have insufficient knowledge or experience to judge questions which may be medically or technically complex, on what basis do you make the decision? Or is it more appropriate to discuss the conflicting views openly and just air the debate more widely?

Health or Healthism?

In their enthusiasm for improving health, there is a danger that health promoters come to see health as the be-all and end-all: as an end in itself, not as a means to the end of enabling people to fulfil their own potential and live life to the full. This ideology of health as the ultimate goal incorporating all life is sometimes called 'healthism'.

The danger is that it may lead to a lack of acceptance that health means different things to different people, shaped by their various values and experiences. Health may become a stereotyped image of the health promoter's own idea of perfection, leading to a prescription of what people should and should not do. This is clearly contrary to the concept that health promotion is about enabling people to increase their *own* control over their health and improve it in ways *they* see fit.

Health Information: an Insensitive Blunderbuss?

All health promotion should be sensitive to the social, ethnic, economic and cultural background of the people it is working with and for. Sadly, this is often not the case. Because of insensitivity, ignorance or the need to produce materials on a large scale for economic reasons, health information, and indeed entire health promotion programmes, are frequently aimed at an 'average' person, or the largest client group. So they often, for example, portray only white people, are only available in English, or assume a level of income above the poverty line. Frequently, it is those with greatest need who are in the minorities and therefore ignored.

There is growing awareness of this issue, but there is still a long way to go before health promotion can truly claim to practise equal opportunities.

To Professionalise or Empower the People?

Health promotion requires special competences, some of which are the subject of this book. It is a whole or part of the work of very many professions, including health, education and community work. As it becomes increasingly specialised, with its own body of knowledge based on research, and its own academic qualifications, there is a danger that health promotion 'experts' will exclude other workers and the public from the business of health promotion.

This would be a sad mistake. Health promotion, as we have often said, is about empowering people to take more control over their own health. Health promotion specialists therefore need to seek to share their knowledge and experience with lay people, to learn from them, and to see them and other workers as valued partners in health promotion endeavours.

Health For Sale?

With scarce resources available for health promotion, and a climate of market economy and income generation, there is an increasing trend towards sponsorship for health promotion activities. One pitfall is the issue of perceived endorsement of products. For example, a health authority could be seen as advocating that patients should take vitamins if it accepted sponsorship of appointment cards printed with the name of the sponsoring vitamin manufacturer.

There is also a move to involve commercial companies in promoting products in a way which also promotes health. For example, food manufacturers may be involved in special promotions for lower fat products. There are dangers here, the most obvious one being that the interests of the company may not be in harmony with those of the health promoter, who will be perceived as endorsing the product. There is also the possibility that the independent credibility of the health promoter is compromised, with the public thinking 'they're just trying to sell me something' instead of perceiving an unbiased, credible health message.

Another pitfall is that health promotion, which should be a fundamental part of the free National Health Service, is seen as a potential money-maker. Basic services, such as health information materials, health teaching and giving advice to commercial companies on health promotion for employees, become subject to charges.

There is a clear need to develop policies and guidelines on these issues.

Making Ethical Decisions

We have identified many areas of ethical concern, and raised difficult issues which do not present easy resolutions or 'right' answers. The following set of questions is designed to help you to think through some of the dilemmas you face, and to make decisions about ethical questions when faced with alternative courses of action.[6]

1. Questions fundamental to decisions about health:

- Will I be creating autonomy in my clients, enabling them to choose freely for themselves and direct their own lives?
- Will I be respecting the autonomy of my clients, whether or not I approve of what they are doing?
- Will I be respecting people equally, with discrimination?
- Will I be serving basic needs before any other wants?

2. Questions about duties and principles:

- Will I be doing good and preventing harm?
- Will I be telling the truth?
- Will I be minimising harm in the long term?
- Will I be honouring promises and agreements?

3. Questions about consequences:

- Will I be increasing individual good?
- Will I be acting for the good of myself?
- Will I be increasing the good of a particular group?
- Will I be increasing the social good?

4. Questions about external considerations:

- What is the most effective and efficient thing to do?
- What is the degree of risk involved?

- Is there a professional code of practice which has bearing on this?
- How certain am I of the evidence of the facts of the matter?
- Are there any disputed facts?
- Are there legal implications, and if so, do I understand them?
- What are the views and wishes of other relevant people?
- Can I justify my actions in terms of the evidence I have before me?

These questions are tools to help clear thinking and moral reasoning. They are not substitutes for personal judgment, but they help you to think through the issue, weigh up the pros and cons and come to a reasoned decision. Not all the questions will be relevant, but they act as a useful checklist. Some questions may reveal that, on the surface, a 'wrong' action is being taken (such as not telling the truth or being discriminatory) but using the checklist ensures that careful consideration is given to it and that it is justified. For example, a painful truth may be withheld from a seriously ill patient, and it may be necessary to discriminate between working with one group of people as opposed to another because there are insufficient resources to work with both.

Exercise—Ethical decisions in health promotion

Case A

The Department of Health (DoH) has issued a circular to all health authorities stating that whooping cough has reached 'epidemic proportions', and urging an immediate campaign at improving uptake of whooping cough vaccination. The Director of Public Health is keen to do so, and instructs the District Health Education Officer (DHEO) to organise the campaign.

The secretary of the Community Health Council (CHC), who claims to represent the consumer's view, has expressed opposition to the proposed campaign. She has recently been involved with the case of a local parent who claims that her child was brain-damaged by whooping cough vaccine, and she reports that the CHC's view is that this proposed local campaign would induce guilt and stress in parents by pressurising them to risk brain damage to their children.

The DHEO faces a dilemma—to run the campaign which the DoH and the Director of Public Health (to whom she is responsible) want, or go along with the views of the CHC who represents her clients?

1. Identify the ethical issues in this situation.
2. What do you think the DHEO should do, and why?

Case B

An Environmental Health Officer (EHO) is chairman of a working group planning a major conference on prevention and education about AIDS. The other members of the working group are a Health Promotion Officer (HPO) and a representative of a prominant local voluntary group working in the AIDS field.

continued on next page

continued

The HPO, with the agreement of the other members of the working group, has secured a promise of a large sum of money donated from a drug company. This will help to meet the expenses of the conference. However, a week before the conference is due to take place, it has been discovered that the drug company has substantial investment in South Africa. (At that time South Africa maintained a policy of apartheid and many people expressed their disapproval with sanctions and boycotts.)

The voluntary group, who oppose all forms of discrimination, say they will withdraw their support for the conference if the money is accepted. The HPO says his health authority has no policy on links with South Africa, and indeed buys large quantities of drugs from this company. Refusal to accept the donation will be very embarrassing for the health authority, and rule out the possibility of future donations for other events. He put a lot of work into obtaining the donation in the first place, and he objects to the imposition of the voluntary group's policy on the other two organisations involved.

The EHO has no strong views either way, but as the Chair he has to ensure that a quick decision is made. The support of both the health authority and the voluntary group is vital to the success of the conference, and the lack of the donation will mean that the conference can go ahead but other planned work will have to be cut in order to fund it.

1. Identify the ethical issues in this situation.
2. What should the Chair decide to do, and why?

Towards a Code of Practice

Many professions have codes of practice which are helpful.[7] We suggest the following as a move towards a code of practice for health promoters.[8]

Relationship to clients

1. It is desirable, wherever possible, to consult clients when planning and evaluating health promotion activities.
2. The promotion of self-esteem and autonomy amongst client groups should be an underlying principle of all health promotion practice.
3. All health promotion practice should encourage people to value others whatever their age, abilities, disabilities or handicaps, race, religion, sex or sexual orientation, and seek to counter discrimination wherever it occurs. Health promoters will support the principle of equal opportunities, taking positive action where this will contribute to a reduction in inequalities in health or health services.

Concern with social and environmental determinants of health

4. All health promotion programmes should be sensitive to the social, economic, racial and cultural framework of the intended client group. Programmes which

focus on specific issues or individuals should always be considered in the context of their wider social, economic and environmental background.

5. All health promotion work should recognise that social, economic and environmental determinants of health are often outside an individual's control, and seek to address these determinants wherever possible.
6. It is desirable for health promotion work to include those methods that encourage the involvement and participation of the public. Empowering people to take more control and responsibility for their own health, so that they have an influence on systems and organisations which affect it, is essential to the pursuit of effective health promotion.

Health promotion practice

7. Appropriate evaluation is an essential component of all health promotion activity, and should be conducted with integrity. This includes giving due recognition to the validity and importance of negative results. Evaluation should, whenever possible, be concerned with input, process and both short-term and long-term outcomes, in order to inform and modify future practice.
8. Health promoters should encourage all services and organisations to consider their health promotion role and to adopt a code of practice. Collaboration between agencies for the promotion of health should be encouraged.
9. Health promoters have a responsibility for ensuring an accurate and appropriate information flow on health issues between the public, professionals, local and national agencies.

Ethical considerations

10. Health promoters will not deliberately withhold services or information which would, in the light of current knowledge, be of benefit to clients. They will endeavour to keep their knowledge of current developments in health promotion up to date.
11. Health promoters will respect the confidentiality of information to which they have access, mindful of the requirements of the law and the best interests of their clients.
12. Health promoters should not undertake health promotion activities which they are not competent to perform.

Exercise—developing a code of practice

Work in small groups of 3 or 4.

Consider the 12 points in the suggested code of practice above.

To what extent do you think you work within this code?

Do you have any suggestions for amendments?

Are there any points you would like to add?

Notes, References and Further Reading

1 Some further reading on philosophy and ethics:

Billington R (1988) *Living Philosophy—an Introduction to Moral Thought*. London: Routledge & Kegan Paul

Doxiadis S (ed) (1987) *Ethical Dilemmas in Health Promotion*. Chichester: Wiley

Doxiadis S (ed) (1990) *Ethics in Health Education*. Chichester: Wiley

Seedhouse D (1988) *Ethics—the Heart of Health Care*. Chichester: Wiley

Downie R S, Fyfe C & Tannahill A (1990) *Health Promotion: Models and Values*. Oxford University Press, Pt 2

Wall A (1989) *Ethics and the Health Service Manger*. King Edward's Hospital Fund for London

2 Some notable articles and readings on models of health education/promotion are:

Burkitt A (1983) Health education. In Clark J & Henderson J (eds) *Community Health*. Edinburgh: Churchill Livingstone, Ch 4

Draper P (1983) Tackling the disease of ignorance. *Self Health*, **1**, 23–25

Catford J & Nutbeam D (1984) Towards a definition of health education and health promotion. *Health Education Journal*, **43**(2 & 3), 38

Tannahill A (1985) What is health promotion? *Health Education Journal*, **44**(4), 167–168

Downie R S, Fyfe C & Tannahill A (1990) *Health Promotion: Models and Values*. Oxford University Press, Pt 1

Tones K, Tilford S & Robinson Y (1990) *Health Education: Effectiveness and Efficiency*. London: Chapman & Hall, Ch 1

French J (1990) Boundaries and horizons, the role of health education within health promotion. *Health Education Journal*, **49**(1), 7–10

3 For discussion about the 'lifestyle approach' and the impact of social factors on health, see:

Graham H (1984) *Women, Health and the Family*. Brighton: Wheatsheaf Books, Ch 12

Blaxter M (1990) *Health and Lifestyles*. London: Tavistock Publications

4 This exercise is based on an idea in the training manual for the Schools Health Education Project 5–13, published by the Health Education Council, London, and reproduced here by kind permission of the Council

5 For a review of the concept of education for self-empowerment, see:

Hopson B & Scally M (1981) *Lifeskills Teaching*. Maidenhead: McGraw-Hill, Ch 3

For a description of the 'self-empowerment model' of health education, see:

Tones K, Tilford S & Robinson Y (1990) *Health Education: Effectiveness and Efficiency*. London: Chapman & Hall, Ch 1

6 The questions in this section are based on the work of Seedhouse, which is recommended for further study:

Seedhouse D (1988) *Ethics—the Heart of Health Care.* Chichester: Wiley. Reproduced by kind permission of John Wiley & Sons Ltd.

7 We suggest that readers make sure they are familiar with the code of practice of their own professional bodies, such as the Health Visitors' Association.

8 This is based on the Society of Health Education and Health Promotion Officers' draft *Principles of Practice* March 1990, and used with the kind permission of the Society.

Chapter 4
Identifying Health Promoters and Their Roles

Summary

The major agents and agencies of health promotion are identified, and their role discussed. They include international and national organisations, the Government, the Health Education Authority, the NHS, local authorities, local groups and many others. An exercise on identifying key local health promoters is included. The chapter ends with suggestions and an exercise on improving the health promotion role.

It is obvious that, to some extent, everyone is a healthy promoter because everyone discusses health matters and gives advice and guidance to others from time to time. This usually happens very informally, for example when parents are reminding children to clean their teeth, or when friends are discussing their experiences. Health promotion may also occur incidentally: for example, the availability of a wide variety of cheap fruit and vegetables in the summer means that it is easier for people to choose a healthy diet. So the greengrocer is unwittingly promoting health. These informal and unplanned sources of health promotion are very significant.

Our aim here, however, is to identify the agents and agencies through which planned, deliberate programmes and policies are channelled.

Agents and Agencies of Health Promotion

Figure 4 indicates the most important agents and agencies of health promotion. Most agents have a variety of health promotion roles—the environmental health departments in local authorities are involved in formal health education, for example, through educating caterers about food handling in kitchens. They are also involved in environmental measures, for example, control of air pollution, and they have important duties related to the enforcement of certain laws, for example, food hygiene regulations and health and safety at work legislation.

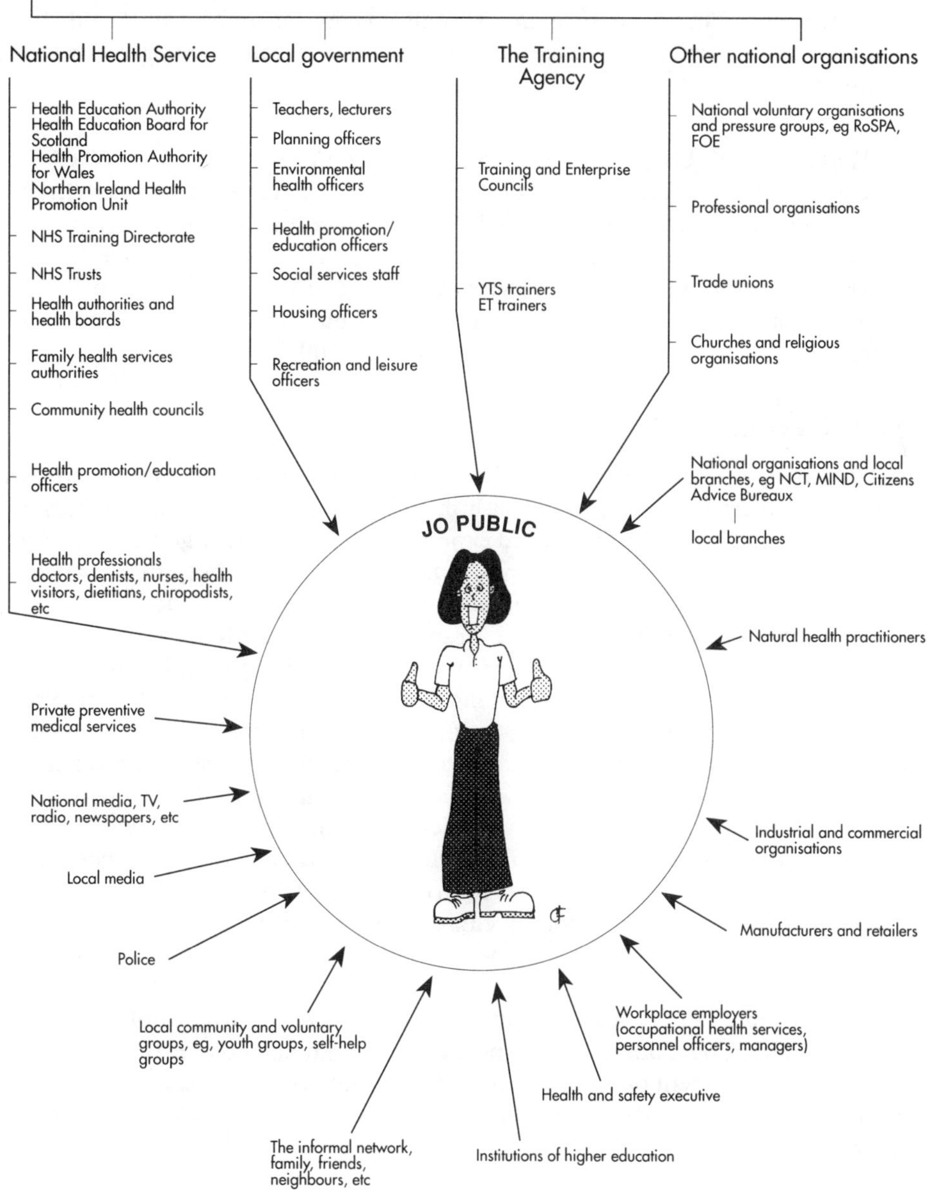
International organisations (World Health Organisation, European Community)
Government (Department of Health, Department of Social Security, Ministry of Agriculture, Fisheries and Food, Department of Education and Science, Central Office of Information, Department of the Environment, Department of Transport, Department of Employment etc)
National Health Service
Health Education Authority
Health Education Board for Scotland
Health Promotion Authority for Wales
Northern Ireland Health Promotion Unit
NHS Training Directorate
NHS Trusts
Health authorities and health boards
Family health services authorities
Community health councils
Health promotion/education officers
Health professionals doctors, dentists, nurses, health visitors, dietitians, chiropodists, etc
Local government
Teachers, lecturers
Planning officers
Environmental health officers
Health promotion/education officers
Social services staff
Housing officers
Recreation and leisure officers
The Training Agency
Training and Enterprise Councils
YTS trainers
ET trainers
Other national organisations
National voluntary organisations and pressure groups, eg RoSPA, FOE
Professional organisations
Trade unions
Churches and religious organisations
National organisations and local branches, eg NCT, MIND, Citizens Advice Bureaux
local branches
JO PUBLIC
Natural health practitioners
Private preventive medical services
National media, TV, radio, newspapers, etc
Local media
Police
Industrial and commercial organisations
Manufacturers and retailers
Local community and voluntary groups, eg, youth groups, self-help groups
Workplace employers (occupational health services, personnel officers, managers)
Health and safety executive
The informal network, family, friends, neighbours, etc
Institutions of higher education

Fig. 4 Agents and agencies in health promotion.

An increasing number of agencies are recognising that they have a role to play in promoting health and this widening ownership of health promotion is helping it to become more effective.

International Organisations

The European Community is increasingly making an impact on health by, for example, setting standards for beach pollution and through directives regulating permitted food additives.

The World Health Organisation's role in 'Health For All by the Year 2000' (HFA) is discussed in the section *Addressing the Determinants of Health* in Chapter One.[1] The WHO European programme is intended to achieve a shift away from a narrow medical view of health towards an understanding of the social influences on health, and it emphasises integration of health services with other related activities such as education, recreation, environmental improvements and social welfare. (This is often referred to as 'intersectoral action' or 'intersectoral collaboration'.)

The Government

In 1991, the UK Government published a significant consultative document which outlined a strategy for improving health in England, with comparable strategies for Wales, Scotland and Northern Ireland expected to follow.[2] Other government departments, notably the Department of Social Security, the Home Office, the Department of Education and Science, the Department of the Environment, the Department of Employment, the Department of the Transport, and the Ministry of Agriculture, Fisheries and Food, also have an interest in, and responsibility for, health promotion, through the impact of legislation, economic and fiscal policies on health. For example, it has been argued that the redistribution of wealth would have a greater effect on health than anything else, short of an improbably large general increase in resources of all kinds.

The structure and organisation of services can also influence health. It remains to be seen how the 1990 National Health Service and Community Care Act will affect the nation's health. It brings about important changes in the way caring services are run; for example, general practitioners are required to provide health checks and are given incentives to run health promotion clinics. One government decision which has received broad support across all parties is to redesignate district medical officers as 'directors of public health'.[3]

The Department of Health sometimes also retains control over public information and health education campaigns on specific issues. An example of this is drug education—the Department of Health initiative on illegal drugs has been widely criticised for setting an inappropriate agenda for this country, where alcohol and legal drugs are bigger problems.[4]

Other National Organisations

The Training Agency (previously the Manpower Services Commission) is the country's national training authority.[5] It operates as an executive agency within the

Employment Department, and reports to the Secretary of State. It is responsible for the development and delivery of government-sponsored vocational education programmes. Training and Enterprise Councils (TECs) are independent companies, directed by local business leaders, with a budget transferred from the Training Agency. There are about 80 TECs in England and Wales with a remit to provide employment training for local businesses and individuals. It includes training for unemployed people so that they have the skills required for local jobs, and youth training under contract with the Government Youth Training Scheme (YTS). Obviously the opportunity and the competence to work are important influences on health, and training may include opportunities for health education.

National Voluntary Organisations and Pressure Groups. There are many national organisations concerned with health promotion, some of which have regional and/or local branches. An example of an organisation which has no local network is The Advisory Council on Alcohol and Drug Education (TACADE). Organisations which have local branches include the National Childbirth Trust (NCT), the National Association for Mental Health (MIND) and the Citizens Advice Bureaux. Most of these organisations produce educational material, and some run training courses for professionals and/or the public. Some organisations primarily act as pressure groups, for example Friends of the Earth.

Professional Associations, such as the British Medical Association (BMA), the United Kingdom Central Council for Nursing, Midwifery and Health Visiting (UKCC), the Royal College of General Practitioners (RCGP) and the Institution of Environmental Health Officers (IEHO) have been influential in policy making, in pressing for legislative changes and in the practice and training of their members in health promotion.

Trade Unions are active in promoting health and safety at work, both by negotiating workplace conditions and through health and safety representatives. *The Health and Safety Executive* also oversees the implementation of health and safety at work legislation.

Commercial and Industrial Organisations have a role in safeguarding the public health. Examples include the Water Boards, refuse removal companies and the transport industries.

Manufacturers and Retailers are increasingly taking the health and safety aspects of their products into account. These include manufacturers of children's wear and toys, food manufacturers, producers of 'green' household products and pharmaceutical companies. Large supermarket chains have made an increasingly wide range of 'healthy' options available to the public. Obviously, all these trends are because of increased consumer demands reflecting heightened awareness of health issues.

The Mass Media such as television, radio, newspapers and magazines undertake health education. This is discussed in more detail in Chapter 15.

Churches and Religious Organisations play an important part in developing values, attitudes and beliefs that affect health. Some provide training in skills, such as meditation, which can improve mental, emotional and spiritual health.

The National Health Service

The Health Education Authority (HEA) (previously the Health Education Council) was established as a special health authority within the NHS in 1987. Under its constitution, it is required to provide information and advice about health directly to members of the public and to support other organisations and people who provide health education to members of the public. It also has an input into wider public health policy through its advice to the Secretary of State for Health. The Authority has published its strategy, which states that the HEA's strategic objective is to ensure that by the year 2000 the people of England are more knowledgable, better motivated and more able to acquire and maintain good health.[6]

The Health Education Board for Scotland is the national agency responsible for health education in Scotland.[7] It is accountable to the Scottish Office Home and Health Department; it organises programmes, projects, training, research and evaluation at national level, and supports health boards and local education authorities with their own health education.

The Northern Ireland Health Promotion Unit and **The Health Promotion Authority for Wales** are bodies performing similar functions for Northern Ireland and Wales.[8]

The NHS Training Directorate is a central training body responsible for providing expertise, advice and guidance on education and training for the NHS. It is an executive arm of the NHS Management Executive and is responsible for ensuring that training in health promotion is included in training schemes for NHS managers and health professions.[9]

District Health Authorities (DHAs) (Health Boards in Scotland and Northern Ireland) and Family Health Services Authorities (FHSAs). As a result of the 1990 NHS and Community Care Act, DHAs and FHSAs now have a 'purchaser' role.[9] They are responsible for purchasing the range of health services required to meet the needs of the population. Services can be purchased from the DHA's own directly-managed units, or from self-governing hospitals and community services, other health authorities, and private health care organisations. The Director of Public Health Medicine is responsible for monitoring the health of the local community and determining health needs. Health service managers also have a facilitative role to play in health promotion and the Institute of Health Services Management has produced an action pack for managers.[10]

The NHS Health Promotion/Education Services are responsible for the provision of consultancy, training, programmes and resources to support health promotion locally. Health promotion education officers liaise with health promotion agents and agencies across the district and beyond, to ensure that activities, wherever initiated, are coordinated and supported.

Primary Health Care Teams. The WHO International Conference on Primary Health Care in Alma-Ata (1978) defined primary health care as:

> '. . . essential health care . . . made universally accessible to individuals and families in the community . . . It forms an integral part both of the country's health system, of which it is the central function and main focus, and of the overall social and economic development of the community.'[12]

Primary health care teams are the first point of people's contact with the National Health Service, bringing health care as close as possible to where people live and work. The role of health promotion in primary health care has been reviewed and government documents emphasise the importance of health education in primary health care settings.[13,14] A useful workbook for primary care teams focuses on their role in the prevention of coronary heart disease and strokes.[15]

In Britain, the work of primary health care is shared by a team. The exact membership of each primary health care team varies but it usually includes:

- the general practitioner—the GP is an independent contractor, and has a contract with a Family Health Services Authority, providing a comprehensive range of medical services for 24 hours a day and seven days a week to those patients in the practice, and to those outside the practice in an emergency. GP contracts set targets for the GP in areas such as immunisation, cervical cytology and screening (health checks) for the elderly, and also set practice budgets. These changes may work for or against the GP's effectiveness in health promotion.[16,17]
- the practice manager/administrator—she is the key person in enabling the smooth running of a practice. She has overall responsibility for ensuring that patients are efficiently, confidentially and caringly received at the practice. She is responsible for appointing receptionists and for arranging in-service training for them. She has an important role in health promotion because she can control access to health information for patients.
- receptionists—the uniqueness and challenges of the receptionist's role have been recognised and courses are now available within colleges of further education. These emphasise the roles of the receptionist in health promotion and provide training in communication skills.
- the practice nurse—she holds clinics for people with chronic conditions such as diabetes, and provides encouragement, education and check-ups. Health promotion clinics such as screening clinics for heart disease, Well Woman and Well Man clinics are also part of her health promotion role. An open learning package for practice nurses has been published by the English National Board for Nursing.[18]
- the district nursing team—this includes the district nursing sister and her team of enrolled nurses and auxiliaries. They are responsible for assessing, implementing and evaluating the nursing needs of patients at home. They have an important role in the education of both patients and their carers.

- the health visitor—health visiting consists of planned activities aimed at the promotion of health and this is achieved through working one-to-one and in groups. The health visitor works with a large network of others concerned with health, sickness and social and educational services.
- the community psychiatric nurse (CPN)—with the implementation of the policy to transfer people with mental health problems out of hospitals and into the community, the community psychiatric nurse is increasingly a member of the Primary Health Care Team. CPNs are involved in all forms of care for the mentally ill and handicapped, and in family and counselling work.
- the community midwife—midwives provide services to all childbearing women during pregnancy and for between 10 and 28 days after the birth of a child. They work closely with the GP and the health visitor in parent education.

Some Primary Health Care Teams also include people with jobs specifically concerned with prevention and health promotion, such as health promotion nurses or primary care facilitators who specialise in helping practices to prevent heart disease.[19]

Other Health Professions. Many other health professions, such as hospital nurses, dentists, hospital and retail pharmacists, opticians and the professions allied to medicine (such as chiropodists and dietitians) have a part to play in health promotion, especially in patient education. However, there is some evidence that loss of control and lack of resources are preventing some professions from making a vital contribution to health promotion.[20]

Community Health Councils. Members can be an influence on district health authority health promotion policies and plans. They may also carry out health education as part of their work with users of health services.

Health Services Outside the NHS

Natural Health Practitioners. An increasing number of natural health practitioners now play a part in promoting health, often through helping people to cope with stress and stress-related conditions. They are often collectively referred to as complementary medicine practitioners.

Private Agencies, some funded through insurance schemes, offer a range of health checks and preventive medical services.

Local Government (County or District Councils)

In the 1980s the 'new' public health was characterised by increasing involvement by local government (often referred to as local authorities) in health issues, which often led to the restructuring of local authority committees and departments.[21] Many local authorities have health committees and full-time health officers responsible for promoting liaison and consultation between all departments of the Local Council, and with other bodies, on matters related to health. Health officers are most frequently based in the Department of Environmental Health, but are sometimes part of a Health Unit directly accountable to the Chief Executive, or based in the Social Services Department. A package produced by the Health Education Authority describes initiatives by Local Authorities.[22]

Environmental Health Officers. The measures necessary to deal with the physical factors in the environment which threaten health, in the widest sense, constitute what is known as 'environmental health'. The organisation of environmental health services is mainly the function of Local Authority Environmental Health Departments. Smaller authorities often combine environmental health with housing or recreation and leisure. National and local legislation gives power to these departments to take advisory and legal action on behalf of people who visit, live or work in an area. The scope for health promotion by these departments is very wide, and constantly growing along with new threats to the environment. Many departments appoint specialist officers to work on specific health issues, such as home safety or promoting fitness.

The Local Education Authority (LEA) has responsibility for health education in schools and further education colleges through the work of teachers and lecturers. Most LEAs have an adviser with specific responsibility for health education, and other staff who provide advice, support and training in health education for teachers.

There have been considerable developments in school health education over the last twenty years: many major curriculum development projects have taken place, resulting in significant progress.[23] The impact on school health education of the National Curriculum (introduced in 1989), the changing role of school governors and the shift of budget-holding responsibilities from local education authorities to schools themselves remains to be evaluated.

Social Services staff, including social workers, staff of residential homes and home helps, are often concerned with improving the health of clients. With the movement towards care in the community for the elderly, the mentally ill and the handicapped, the role of Social Services Departments in promoting the health of these vulnerable groups is increasing.[24]

Many other local authority staff have a role in health promotion, such as recreation and leisure officers, housing officers and youth and community workers.

Other Local Organisations and Groups

There are numerous individuals and groups at local level who help to promote particular aspects of health. Some notable ones are:

Institutions of Higher Education. Polytechnics and universities are responsible for the basic professional training of the professions with health promotion roles. They are also increasingly involved in postbasic and continuing education for health promoters, including running Health Education Certificate Courses.[25] The Open University has been very active, both in developing degree courses in health, especially useful to professionals without a first degree, and in producing community education material on health issues for the general public.[26]

Local Voluntary and Community Groups. A huge range of local voluntary and community groups exist, many of which undertake educational work on health matters. Patients associations, self-help groups, environmental action groups and youth groups are just a few examples. (Community-based work in health promotion is discussed in Chapter 12.)

Employers can be active in developing health-promoting policies and conditions in the workplace. Personnel officers and occupational health staff, in particular, are vital to the implementation of workplace policies and in promoting the well-being of staff.

Police and Probation Officers. The police protect the public from crime and violence, take action to prevent misuse of drugs and alcohol and help to ensure road safety. Prison officers and probation officers are involved in the health and well-being of prisoners and their families.

The next exercise is designed to help you to identify the health promotion agents and agencies which are important for your work. There is much to gain by having good local knowledge of other people you can work with or refer people to.

Exercise—What's on your patch? Finding out about your local agents and agencies in health promotion

Think of the geographical 'patch' where you work, and identify its boundaries as clearly as you can. For example, this could be the area served by a GP practice, the catchment area served by a hospital/health service or the geographical patch defined as your responsibility as an environmental health officer or community worker.

Identify as many health promotion agents and agencies on your patch as you can, using Figure 4 and the list above as a checklist.

It is likely that you will know some of them very well and others not at all. Identify any which it would be helpful to know more about, and plan to find out about them.

If there are some that you know nothing about, such as the community groups which exist on your patch, identify people who do know about them (such as local health visitors, health education/promotion departments) and plan to find out more.

The Informal Network

Finally, as we mentioned in the opening paragraph of this chapter, it is essential to remember that the whole informal network of family, friends and neighbours is of great significance in shaping people's health beliefs and behaviour and in providing healthy living conditions.[27]

Improving Your Health Promotion Role

A number of factors affect the development of the health promotion role of professionals. The need for improved training has been recognised.[28] One of the difficulties this raises is how to fit more into the already overcrowded curriculum of basic professional training courses. Partial solutions might be to identify the core competences needed by health promoters and to integrate skills training into other aspects of professional training, on the basis that these skills are transferrable to health promotion work.

Postbasic courses, such as Health Education Certificate courses, and postgraduate diplomas and masters degrees in health education and health promotion are increasingly available, often in a range of learning modes such as full-time, part-time, college-based or open learning.[29] There is an urgent need to look at credit accumulation related to diploma level and masters degree courses so that students with relevant certificates can be awarded credits towards higher-level courses. The use of open learning for more components of professional development could also be explored. By minimising the time students are 'off the job', managers could be encouraged to release staff for training.

A problem for students is that they use trained professionals as examples to follow (role models), but research shows that trained professionals themselves may not have the necessary skills.[30] This is particularly true of skills in networking, facilitating, marketing and political skills, which have not traditionally been included in professional training.

Some professionals have too narrow a concept of health and what is meant by health promotion and by health education; therefore they may only use individual behaviour change approaches and fail to take advantage of opportunities for using alternative or complementary approaches. Lack of knowledge about which approaches to health promotion are likely to be effective in different circumstances is also a problem, so ineffective methods continue to be used.

Furthermore, the health promotion and health education needs of the professionals themselves may not have been met. Although they may be exhorted to be a good example they are often not given the help they need to make health choices and carry these through.

In addition, resource constraints may hinder the professions from achieving their potential in health promotion. There is an acknowledged shortage of staff in the Professions Allied to Medicine.[31] There is evidence that work overload is forcing health visitors to spend more of their time coping with child abuse crises with less time available for long-term health promotion work.[32] The need for education and training of policy makers and managers has been highlighted.[33]

On the positive side, there is ample evidence that patients want more information and welcome opportunistic health education from, for example, general practitioners.[34] Evidence concerning the effectiveness of professionals in promoting health is growing[35] and there is also evidence that training can make them even more effective.[36] For example, a training course on communication skills for nurses has been developed and the success of this project has led to a multiprofessional initiative for nurses, doctors, physiotherapists and occupational therapists.[37,38]

In connection with health visiting, pioneering work has been carried out to investigate how health visitors can work in different ways—for example with groups and communities instead of concentrating on individuals.[39] The professional associations have played an important part in updating concepts about the health promotion role of their members.[40]

In summary, some strategies have proved very useful in improving the role of professionals in health promotion. But overall education and training for professionals remains an underdeveloped area, particularly the training of policy-makers and managers, and training in the skills of networking, facilitation, marketing and influencing policy and practice.

The following exercise is designed to help you to identify factors which help and hinder you in carrying out health promotion work, and what you might do to improve the situation.

Exercise—What helps and hinders your health promotion work?

This exercise is designed to help you to identify helping and hindering forces in your own situation.

In a stable system, the forces for producing changes are equally offset by forces opposed to change. It is essential to pinpoint all the possible helping and hindering forces, so that you can take steps to increase the power of helping forces, and decrease the power of the hindering forces. The disruption of the balance results in progress towards change.

For your own situation:

- make a list of *forces which help you* in your health promotion work;
- make a list of *forces which hinder you* in your health promotion work;
- identify *ways of increasing the helping forces*
- identify *ways of decreasing the hindering forces*

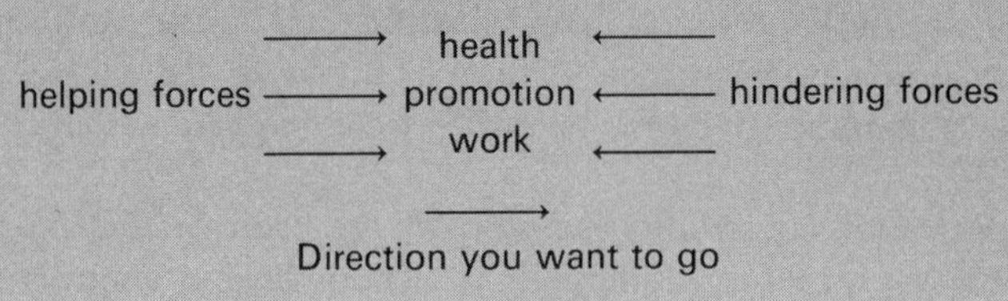

Notes, References and Further Reading

1 WHO Regional Office for Europe (1985) *Targets for Health for All.* Denmark: WHO, Scherfigsveg 8, DK-2100 Copenhagen

2 Secretary of State for Health (1991) *The Health of the Nation: a Consultative Document for Health in England.* London: HMSO

3 Committee of Enquiry into the Future Development of the Public Health Function (1988) *Public Health in England*. London: HMSO

4 See, for example:

Whitehead M & Adams L (1989) Time for a new agenda. *Health Service Journal*, (5th October), 1220

5 The Training Agency, Moorfoot, Sheffield, S1 4PQ. Telephone: 0742 753275

6 Health Education Authority (1989) *Strategic Plan 1990–95*. London: HEA

Health Education Authority, Hamilton House, Mabledon Place, London WC1H 9TX. Telephone: 071 383 3833

7 *Health Education Board for Scotland*, Health Education Centre, Woodburn House, Canaan Lane, Edinburgh EH10 4SG. Telephone: 031 447 8044

8 *Northern Ireland Health Promotion Unit*, The Beeches, 12 Hampton Manor Drive, Belfast BT7 3EN. Telephone: 0232 644811

The Health Promotion Authority for Wales, Brunel House, 8th Floor, 2 Fitzalan Road, Cardiff CF1 1EB. Telephone: 0222 472472

9 For example, *Health PICKUP* is a modular training programme to develop the non-clinical skills of qualified professionals in the health service. The modules include skills training in some of the core competences required by health promoters: managing yourself and your work, helping others to learn and multidisciplinary teamworking.

Managing Health Services is an open learning course designed to meet the needs of health service managers, commissioned by the NHSTA and produced by the Open University in collaboration with the Institute of Health Services Management (IHSM). Book 10 discusses illness prevention.

NHS Training Directorate (previously the NHS Training Authority), St Bartholomews Court, 18 Christmas Street, Bristol BS1 5BT. Telephone: 0272 291029

10 Department of Health (1989) *Working for Patients*. White Paper (CM555). London: HMSO

For a concise account of the development of the NHS from 1948 to the NHS review in 1989 see:

Leathard A (1990) *Health Care Provision: Past, Present and Future*. London: Chapman & Hall

11 Institute of Health Services Management in conjunction with the Faculty of Community Medicine (December 1988) *Health For All—A Management Action Pack*. London: IHSM

See also:

Disken S (1990) Health for all and all for one. *Health Service Journal* (10th May), 691. This article describes the activities of the IHSM Health for All Group.

12 World Health Organisation (1978) Report on the Primary Health Care Conference, Alma-Ata. Geneva: World Health Organisation

13 Stott N C H (1986) The role of health promotion in primary health care. *Health Promotion*, **1**(1), 49–52

14 DHSS (1986) *Primary Health Care, an Agenda for Discussion*. London: HMSO

DHSS (1987) Promoting Better Health, *The Government's Programme for Improving Primary Health Care*. White Paper (CM249). London: HMSO

15 Tudor Hart J & Stilwell B (1988) *Prevention of Coronary Heart Disease and Strokes: a Workbook for Primary Care Teams*. London: Faber & Faber

16 See for example:

Moran G (1989) Public health at risk. *Health Service Journal* (1st June), 668–669

17 For a useful review of the role of the GP in health education, see:

Roland M O (1989) What is a GP's role in health education? *Journal of the Institute of Health Education*, **27**(4), 172–178

18 English National Board for Nursing (ENB) (1989) *Health Promotion in Primary Health Care, an Open Learning Package for Practice Nurses*. Learning Materials Design

19 Fullard E, Fowler G & Gray M (1987) Promoting prevention in primary care: controlled trial of low-technology, low-cost approach. *British Medical Journal*, **294** (25th April)

20 See for example:

Lyne P & Stone S (1990) Talent waiting to be tapped. *Health Service Journal*, (12th April), 550–551

21 See for example:

Health Education Authority/Oxford City Council (1988) *Oxford—a Healthy City Strategy*. London: HEA

22 Health Education Authority (1991) *Promoting Health—Local Authorities in Action*. London: HEA.

23 For more about health education in schools and with young people see:

David K & Williams T (eds) (1987) *Health Education in Schools*. London: Harper & Row

National Curriculum Council (1990) *Curriculum Guidance 5: Health Education*. York: National Curriculum Council, 15–17 New Street, York YO1 2RA

Nutbeam D, Haglund B, Farley P & Tillgren P (eds) (1990) *Youth Health Promotion: From Theory to Practice in School and Community*. London: Forbes Publications

For a discussion of recent trends in school health education, see:

Whitehead M (1989) *Swimming Upstream—Trends and Prospects in Education for Health.* Research Report 5. London: King's Fund Institute, Section 2

Significant early curriculum projects were:

Schools Council/Health Education Council Project:

5–8-year-olds *All About Me.* (1977) London: Nelson
9–13-year-olds *Think Well.* (1977) London: Nelson
13–18-year-olds (1982) London: Forbes

These have been identified by many as an important influence in putting health education on the agenda in schools, and in laying the groundwork for the development of subsequent school projects.

There is now a large and growing number of curriculum development materials, teachers' guides and classroom materials for health education in schools: these cover both broad health education programmes and work in specific subject areas such as alcohol, drugs, smoking, dental health, preventing heart disease and preving child abuse. There are materials for primary, secondary and special schools, and colleges, and also for use during initial teacher training, in-service training of teachers, and for use with school governors.

For details, contact:

- the Health Education/Health Promotion Department in your local district health authority or health board
- the Health Education Authority (for address see Note 5 above) who produce lists of resources
- the Advisory Council on Alcohol and Drug Education (TACADE) produces material and runs in-service training. Address: 1 Hulme Place, The Crescent, Salford M5 4QA

The importance of the whole school in providing a health promoting environment through a 'health promoting school' is highlighted in a SHEG report:

Scottish Health Education Group/Scottish Consultative Council on the Curriculum (1989) *Promoting Good Health—Proposals for Action.* Edinburgh: SHEG

24 Department of Health (1989) *Caring for People: Community Care in the Next Decade and Beyond.* White Paper (CM849). London: HMSO

25 Health Education Certificate courses for professionals are one-day-a-week, day-release courses lasting for one academic year; there are about 50 of these in polytechnics and colleges of further and higher education in the UK. For details write to the Health Education Authority (see Note 5 above for the address), or sister organisations in Scotland, Wales and Ireland (see Notes 5 and 6 above). The HEA will also give details of diploma and masters degree courses in health education and health promotion.

The Health Education Authority has also sponsored and funded a Certificate in Health Education Open Learning Project, in the Department of Education at Keele University. This is aimed at students wishing to proceed to the Certificate in Health Eduction, but for whom attendance at a college-based course is not possible. For further details contact the Project Director,

Department of Education, University of Keele, Staffordshire ST5 5BG. Telephone: 0782 621111.

26 For details of the Open University Community Education materials, contact:

Department of Community Education, The Open University, Walton Hall, Milton Keynes, MK7 6AA. Telephone: 0908 653743

27 For further reading on the influence of informal networks on health beliefs and behaviour, see:

Blaxter M & Paterson E (1982) *Mothers and Daughters: A Three-generational Study of Health Attitudes and Behaviour*. London: Heinemann

Graham H (1984) *Women, Health and the Family*. Brighton: Wheatsheaf Books, Ch 11

28 For example, the United Kingdom Central Council for Nursing, Midwifery and Health Visiting has emphasised the need for improved training in health promotion in Project 2000. See:

UKCC (1986) *Project 2000: a New Preparation for Practice*. London: United Kingdom Central Council

The Scottish Health Education Group (SHEG) (now Health Education Board for Scotland, HEB) set up a project to develop curriculum material on health education in nursing:

SHEG (1986) *The Basic Curriculum Project*. Edinburgh: Scottish Health Education Group

The Health Education Authority has funded a number of projects to research and support the role of professionals: these include general practitioners, nurses, environmental health officers and the professions allied to medicine. See, for example:

Lyne P A (1984) *Just Repairing the Damage? Health Education and the Professions Allied to Medicine—a Report on a Preliminary Study*. London: Health Education Council

29 See Note 23 above.

Diploma and masters courses have been developed since the early 1970s in colleges and universities around the country, some with initial financial support from the Health Education Authority

30 See, for example:

Faulkner A *et al.* (1985) *Communication in Nurse Education: Survey of Schools of Nursing*. Research Project 1982–85. London: Health Education Council

31 Independent Commission into Occupational Therapy (1989) *Occupational Therapy: an Emerging Profession in Health Care*. London: Duckworth

This reported that more than a quarter of funded posts for basic-grade occupational therapists were vacant in March 1988. This shortage is troubling in the light of the increasing numbers of elderly people in the population and the move to community care of mentally ill and mentally handicapped people.

These shortages are also aggravated by worries about future recruitment because of the fall in the number of 18-year-olds.

32 Sharma A & Sunderland R (1988) Increasing medical burden of child abuse. *Archives of Diseases in Childhood*, **63**, 172–175

33 See, for example:

Ginnerty P, Wilde J & Black M (1989) Participation in practice: an example from Belfast. In Martin C & McQueen D (eds) *Readings for a New Public Health*. Edinburgh University Press

34 See, for example:

Sullivan D (1988) Opportunistic health promotion: do patients like it? *Journal of Royal College of GPs*, **38**, 24–25

35 For example, a randomised controlled trial to determine the effectiveness of advice from GPs (who had received special training) to heavy drinkers found that alcohol consumption was reduced significantly in the experimental group compared with the controls. The study concluded that if the results were applied to the whole of the UK, health education by GPs could each year reduce to moderate levels the alcohol consumption of 250,000 men and 67,000 women who currently drink to excess. See:

Wallace P *et al* (1988) Randomised controlled trial of GP interventions in patients with excessive alcohol consumption. *British Medical Journal*, **297**, 663–668

36 For example, a study of nurses' attempts to help their patients give up smoking found that 17 per cent of the experimental group who were followed up after a year had given up smoking, compared with 8 per cent of the controls. The experimental group of nurses had taken part in a two-day training programme to introduce them to health promotion approaches in nursing. See:

Macleod-Clark J *et al* (1987) *Helping Patients and Clients to Stop Smoking Phase 2: Assessing the Effectiveness of the Nurse's Role*. Research Report No. 19. London: Health Education Authority

37 See Macleod-Clark J *et al* (1987), Note 36, above

38 Macleod-Clark J *et al* (1987) Helping nurses develop their education role, a framework for training. *Nurse Education Today*, 7, 63–68

39 See Drennan V (1986) *Working in a Different Way*. Health Education Department, Paddington & North Kensington Health Authority, and Drennan (1988) *Health Visitors and Groups: Politics and Practice*. Oxford: Heinemann Nursing

40 For example, the Health Visitors Association has reviewed the roles of health visitors and school nurses in:

Health Visitors Association (1987) *Health Visiting and School Nursing Reviewed*. London: HVA

It states that:

> The health visitor, by promoting health and health policies, empowers people to take responsibility for health as individuals, families and communities, and thereby helps to prevent and minimise the effects of disease, dysfunction and disability.
>
> The school nurse, by promoting health and health education in the school environment, works to minimise a child's obstacles to learning and to maximise children's potential for living.

The Institution of Environmental Health Officers has supported the evolution of the new public health. For a view of the role of environmental health officers, see:

Bassett W (ed) (1990) *Clay's Environmental Health Officers Handbook*. London: Chapman & Hall

PART II

MOVING FROM THEORY TO PRACTICE

Introduction

Part II has three purposes.

- To provide guidance on how you can identify the views and needs of the clients/users/receivers of health promotion, and set priorities for your work.
- To provide guidance on how you can plan and evaluate your health promotion work.
- To provide guidance on how you can organise and manage your work in order to be effective and efficient.

Chapter Five considers what we mean by a 'need' for health promotion and describes the sources of information required to identify the needs of a community, a group, or an individual person. Guidelines are provided on how to assess needs and set priorities.

Chapter Six identifies a seven-stage planning and evaluation cycle, which will help you to clarify what you are trying to achieve, what you are going to do, and how you will know whether you are succeeding.

Chapter Seven provides guidance on managing health promotion, concentrating on key aspects such as co-ordination and teamwork, participating in meetings, report writing, managing paperwork and managing time.

Chapter 5
Identifying Health Promotion Needs and Priorities

Summary

An analysis of the concept of need is followed by a section discussing four factors to consider when identifying health promotion needs (the scope, reactive/proactive choices, putting the user at the centre and adopting a marketing philosophy), and an exercise on the 'user-friendliness' of services. The next section on finding and using health information identifies varieties and sources of information. A framework for assessing health promotion needs follows, with a case study and an exercise. The final section focuses on setting priorities, and includes exercises on analysing the reasons for health promotion priorities and on setting priorities.

Identifying the people who are intended to benefit from health promotion activities is a complex process which takes place at many levels, from global and national to the level of local communities, groups, families and individuals. These people may be referred to as 'users', by which we mean those who use health promotion *services*, such as prevention clinics, maternity services and pest control services. In some cases people 'receive' help rather than 'use' it, for example receiving advice, information or health education. Alternatively, people may be called 'consumers', 'customers', 'clients', or, of course, 'patients' if they are receiving preventive medical services. Sometimes *potential* users are as important to identify as current users, because a service may not be accessible or attractive to some groups of users. Positive action may be necessary for some people to get the same out of existing services as everybody else.

Going one stage further and identifying people's *needs*, and prioritising them, is also a complex and difficult process. There is a bottomless pit of needs, and only finite resources available to meet them, so difficult choices have to be made.

At global, national and regional level, the assessment of health promotion needs, and the formulation of policies and plans to meet those needs, are part of the work of WHO, government departments, the Health Education Authority in England and its equivalents in Scotland, Wales and Northern Ireland, and regional health authorities, among others. At district health authority or health board level, it is the responsibility of those charged with purchasing health care for their population. The Director of Public Health Medicine usually has a key role. At local authority level it is usually the responsibility of a health committee, with its membership drawn from local councillors and attended by senior officers from a range of departments. Increasingly, health authorities, local authorities and other agencies are undertaking joint information-gathering related to health promotion needs, and developing joint plans.[1] Consideration of identifying needs at these larger-scale levels is outside the scope of this book—our concern is with the level of work undertaken by health promoters working with individual clients, families, groups and communities.[2]

Before looking further at how we can meet the needs of the users and receivers of health promotion, it is worth considering first what may be meant by a *need.*

Concepts of Need

It is useful to think of four kinds of need.[3]

Normative Need

Normative need is need defined by an expert or professional according to her own standards; falling short of those standards means that there is a need. For example, a dietitian may identify a certain level of nutritional knowledge as the desirable standard for her client and she defines a need for nutrition education if her client's knowledge does not reach that standard. This normative need is based on the value judgments of professional experts, which may lead to two problems: one is that expert opinion may vary over what is the acceptable standard, and the other that the values and standards of the experts may differ from those of their clients. Some normative needs, such as food hygiene regulations, are prescribed by law.

Felt Need

Felt need is the need in which people identify what they *want*. For example, a pregnant woman may feel the need for and therefore want information about childbirth. Felt needs may be limited or inflated by people's awareness and knowledge about what could be available, so, for example, people will not have a felt need for knowing their blood cholesterol level if they have never heard that such a thing is possible.

Expressed Need

Expressed need is what people say they need; in other words, it is felt need which has been turned into an expressed request or *demand*. The demand for exercise classes and fitness testing are examples of expressed need. It is worth noting that not all felt need is turned into expressed need. Lack of opportunity, motivation or assertiveness could all prevent the expression of a felt need. Lack of demand should not be equated with lack of felt need.

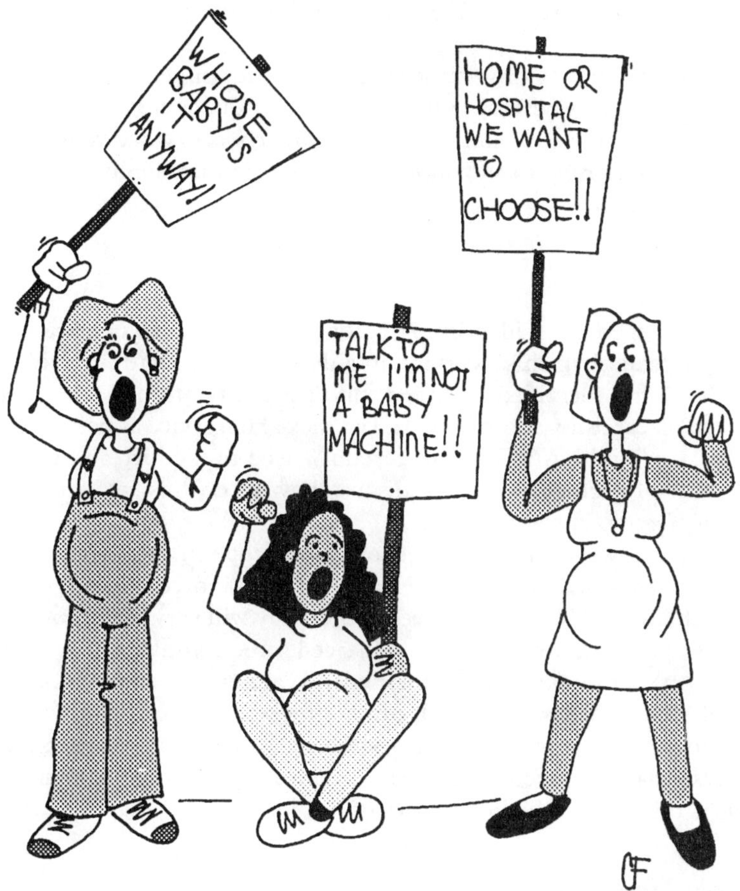
WHOSE BABY IS IT ANYWAY!
TALK TO ME I'M NOT A BABY MACHINE!!
HOME OR HOSPITAL WE WANT TO CHOOSE!!
CF

Expressed need is felt need turned into demand

Expressed needs may conflict with a professional's normative needs. For example, a patient may express a need for a considerable amount of information on his medical condition, and this may be far more than a nurse is able or willing to give. The converse may also happen, with the nurse wishing to tell the patient far more than he wants to know.

Comparative Need

Comparative need for health promotion is defined by comparison between similar groups of clients, some of whom are in receipt of health promotion and some are not. Those who are not are then defined as being in need. For example, if Company A has health policies about smoking at work and provides 'healthy' food choices in the staff dining room and Company B does not, it could be said that there is a comparative need for health promotion in Company B.

To summarise: *Need, like beauty, is in the eye of the beholder.*[4]

Identifying Health Promotion Needs

How does a worker in health promotion set about identifying the needs of people? We identify four key areas it is useful to think about first: the boundaries of your job, the balance of your work between being *reactive* and *proactive*, to what extent you put your clients first, and the usefulness of adopting a marketing philosophy. We address each of these in turn.

The Scope

For some workers the task of identifying needs has already been done to some extent. For example, a dental hygienist working in a dental surgery with individual patients already has the clearly identified task of educating her patients in oral hygiene. But she may want to think carefully about how she can make her service as person-centred and user-friendly as possible. And she will certainly need to identify and respond to the individual needs of each patient. (We discuss how to do this in Part 3: *Developing Competence in Health Promotion.*)

Other workers, however, have more choice and scope in the range of health promotion activities they can undertake. Health visitors and community workers may have considerable scope, but their degree of autonomy will vary according to the policy of their managers. All health promoters will need some competency in being responsive to the health promotion needs of their clients, and will need to be clear about the boundaries of their work: which health promotion activities are within their remit to undertake, and which are not, however desirable they may be. For example, a family planning nurse may be asked to undertake education work with young people in schools, but is this within the boundaries of her job?

Reactive or Proactive?

It is useful to make an initial distinction between being *reactive* and *proactive* when identifying needs. Being reactive means responding (ie. reacting) to the needs and demands which other people make. Pressure from vested interest groups and the media may introduce bias into how needs are perceived, and produce pressure to react. Being proactive means taking the initiative and deciding oneself on the area of work to be done. It may include saying 'no' to the demands of other people if these do not fit existing policies and priorities.

Being reactive or proactive can be related to the approaches to health promotion which were discussed in Chapter Three. Using a client-directed approach means being reactive to consumers' expressed needs, whereas using a medical or behaviour-change approach probably means being proactive. This is particularly true of preventive medical interventions such as immunisation campaigns. In practice, there is usually a balance to be struck between being reactive and proactive.

Putting Users' Needs First

Whose needs should come first—the users' or the providers'? There may be conflict between the two; for example, users may want a family planning service open on

Saturdays but providers are unable to do so because of difficulties of getting staff to work at weekends. However, we identify several trends which have emphasised putting the views and needs of users at the centre of the provision of health promotion.[5]

- The emphasis on the user as a unique individual person.
- The trend towards professionals working in partnership with lay people.
- The emphasis on improving the availability of, and access to, services which promote health, for example, leisure and recreational services, preventive health services.
- The trend towards a client-centred approach to health education, with self-empowerment of the client the key aim.
- The trend towards more user participation in the planning and evaluation of health promotion activities.

Two other trends which play a part are the growth of the wider consumer movement since the 1960s, and the influence on service provision of market models in the late 1980s. An interest in the techniques of commercial enterprise is now widespread amongst public sector managers. Health service managers are recommended to use market research, among other methods, to find out about the experience and perceptions of patients and the community.[6]

One of the most important ways of making activities more responsive to users and receivers is to give them more control over what happens to them. There is an increasing number of local authority and health authority initiatives that aim to give users more choice.[7]

Adopting a Marketing Approach[8]

We referred to the growth of the consumer movement in health services and market models above; 'marketing' is a term frequently used in relation to health promotion. Marketing is often associated solely with commercial businesses and making profits, and with the activities of sales and advertising. How, then, does it relate to health promotion and, more specifically, to the question of identifying needs?

Health promoters usually work in the public or voluntary sectors, and are not generally required to make profits, and so are different from commercial enterprises. But the health promoter could be more effective and efficient through adopting a marketing approach. The fact that health is obviously a 'good thing', which therefore does not need a 'hard sell', and that health promotion services often emphasise person-to-person involvement, has tended to convince health promoters that they are in touch with their clients/users and that marketing may have nothing more to offer. However, there is increasing recognition that this is not so.

Although the phrase 'the customer is always right' originated in the service industries, there are many cases where this is patently not practised. For example, people are placing an increasing value on their time, and resent it if they are kept waiting because the professional's time appears to be more valuable than their own.

What would 'adopting a marketing approach' mean in the context of health promotion? We start by suggesting the following definition of marketing:

Marketing, in the context of health promotion, is the management skill of identifying opportunities for satisfying consumers'/clients' requirements and, by doing so, maximising the protection and/or improvement of their health.[9]

So the output is health, not profits. Fundamentally, marketing is an attitude of mind. It is about identifying consumer needs and satisfying them in the most efficient way, so that the maximum output is achieved in terms of people's health. Through adopting this approach, health promotion activities can benefit from greater effectiveness and efficiency, and from improved consumer satisfaction. In certain circumstances this may involve using specific marketing techniques, such as market research. It also means being much more responsive to the consumers' needs and wants, tailoring services to these rather than to the providers' ideas of what they think people should have. A marketing approach means making services user-friendly, and the following exercise provides a checklist to assess how user-friendly your health promotion services are.

Exercise—How user-friendly are your services?[10]

Below is a list of ten factors which may affect how users view the services you offer. Rate each service you offer on each factor using a scale from 1 (very poor) to 5 (excellent). The maximum score is 50. How do your services measure up?

Availability of service—do the times suit the user?
Accessibility—easy access by public transport? Easy car parking?
Quality of service—what are the standards, reliability, results?
Speed of service—do appointments keep to schedule?
Friendly service—a warm, welcoming atmosphere, continuity of relationships?
Good environment—safe, warm, clean, comfortable?
Information about the service—is it widely available, inviting, accurate, easy to understand?
Reputation of the service—do local people rate the service highly?
Attitudes—is there an understanding and acknowledgment of the user's circumstances and feelings?
Responsiveness of the service—is the service relevant to local people, does it reach all potential groups of users, are suggestions encouraged and complaints handled sensitively?

We now return to the central questions: how can needs for health promotion be identified, and once identified, what criteria can the health promoter use to decide whether, and how, to respond?

Finding and Using Information

The starting point for defining health promotion needs is *information* of various kinds from a range of sources. If information is being gathered on a local area for the first time, it would be helpful to share the work, and the findings, with colleagues. Health visitors may have done a neighbourhood profile as part of their training. The local health authority health promotion department may have gathered information. In any case, gathering and up-dating this information is a continuing project for every health promoter and sharing the burden makes sense. Working with colleagues must go hand in hand with developing good links with the community, in order to gear health promotion more effectively towards active participation of users and receivers.

We will now look at the major kinds of information and how this may help to identify health promotion needs.

Epidemiological Data

Epidemiology is the study of the distribution and determinants of disease in communities; epidemiological data indicate how many people are affected by a health problem, how many people die from a particular health problem, and who are most at risk (for example, men or women? which age groups? which social class? which occupation? which geographical area? fat or thin people? smokers or non-smokers? sedentary or active people?).

Mortality and morbidity data are collected nationally, and some data are also available on a regional and local basis. (Mortality data are concerned with causes of death; morbidity data are concerned with types of illness and disability.) Mortality data are derived from death certificates; morbidity data are derived from a wide range of sources, including general practice records, hospital records, sickness absence certificates, child health records, returns of notifiable diseases, disability registers and many others. In addition, surveys such as the government's General Household Survey, and surveys carried out for research purposes provide a considerable amount of health information.

The District Health Authority information department should be able to provide a copy of the Annual Health Report for the health district and mortality and morbidity data (such as admission rates for particular conditions) for the district as a whole and for smaller areas such as electoral wards. It might be helpful to compare district and electoral ward data (for a neighbourhood) on, for example:

- the major causes of death;
- the key causes of childhood admission to hospital;
- the main conditions for which adults are admitted to hospital.

Detailed discussion of the sources and limitations of epidemiological data is outside the scope of this book, and further reading is suggested.[11] The important point to make here is that epidemiological data provide essential information on the health of the population, the causes and risk factors related to ill-health, and consequently, the potential for prevention and health promotion.

Socioeconomic Data

The planning or information departments of local councils should be able to help with information about housing, employment, social class and social/leisure/recreation/ shopping facilities. Many produce summaries of census data. It might be helpful to compare district/borough/city and electoral ward data on, for example:

- unemployment;
- household amenities;
- social class;
- head of household born outside Britain.

It is advisable to ask for figures which are as full and recent as possible. Much data are obtained from the census which takes place every ten years, and information sought in the early 1990s is likely to go back to the 1981 census. This did not, for example, include ethnic monitoring; 1991 census data, when available, will be more helpful.

By setting illness alongside socioeconomic data, you may be able to see particular patterns of inequalities in health in your area. The Annual Report of your District Health Authority or reports from your local authority may look at this issue in detail.

Professional Views

The views of fellow health promoters reflect experience and perceptions accumulated over the years which it would be foolish to ignore. What do other workers in the area, such as teachers, youth workers, social workers, GPs, health visitors, district nurses, environmental health officers, police officers, community workers and religious leaders, consider to be the major health concerns?

Public Views

There are several methods of obtaining the views of the public. These range from informal discussions/interviews to large-scale surveys using questionnaires or in-depth interview techniques.[12] A number of attempts have been made to classify the various ways of involving users in the planning of services.[13] Identifying priority groups and thinking clearly about them will influence the choice of methods used to contact and involve them.

It is better to begin with the characteristics of the groups and then design the best approach. For instance, how large are the relevant groups? Do they have particular age, class or ethnic structures? What makes it a 'group' (geography, membership, current use of services and facilities)? Are the members of the group mobile? Do they have easy access to transport facilities? What times of day are they likely to be available for meetings? Be absolutely clear about what sort of relationship you are proposing to have with local groups and individuals. (This is discussed in detail in Chapter 12, *Working with Communities*.) For example, if the plan is simply to establish consultation mechanisms, there may be hostility if local people have played a stronger role in other circumstances.

The groups involved may include the Community Health Council (established by the 1973 NHS Act to represent the user's voice in the NHS), local voluntary organisations and community groups such as self-help groups, black and other minority ethnic groups, pensioners' clubs, tenants' associations, and a variety of local advisory groups or planning subcommittees, in addition to groups of key clients such as mothers. Gathering views *informally* is a useful dipstick but there are, of course, problems about the accuracy and representativeness of subjective information. However, this subjective data can usefully feed into the wider framework.

One of the most powerful ways of finding out what it is really like for users is to experience a service at first hand.[14] This can result in individual workers radically changing their working practices but it may not always be possible to translate this experiment into general changes in the way services are delivered.

You may want to consider undertaking some first-hand research, but first think about how much time and money it will take. Will the results justify the costs? If you still think it is worth doing, who could do it? If it is on a very small scale you could perhaps undertake it yourself, maybe in collaboration with some colleagues.

Local Media

The opinions and data collected will provide you with a picture at a particular point of time. Monitoring local radio, TV and papers will give a view of any major changes in the community as they happen. All this adds to the profile of local information which is building up, providing a basis for planning health promotion.

Assessing Health Promotion Needs

The assessment of health promotion needs can be approached systematically by asking a series of key questions. The answers will help you to decide whether to respond to a particular need, and if so, how.

What sort of need is it?

Is it a normative, felt, expressed or comparative need? In a parent education class, for example, what kind of need is being met: the *normative* needs decided by the health professional, the *felt* or *expressed* needs of the parents or *comparative* needs decided after looking at what was available elsewhere?

Who decided that there is a need?

Whose decision is it: the health promoter's, the client's or both? Sometimes the answer to this question is not immediately obvious because the need has emerged after discussion between the health promoter and client. People do not always know what they need or want, because their awareness and knowledge of the possibilities is limited. The health promoter may help by raising awareness and knowledge of health issues; in this way she may create a demand (an *expressed* need) for health promotion. For example, the public's demand for wider availability of restaurants with a no-smoking policy only came after health promoters had raised awareness of the hazards of passive smoking. The ideal situation is a joint decision by clients and health promoters.

What are the grounds for deciding that there is a need?

Is there any evidence of need in the form of objective data, such as facts and figures? If *local* data are not available, has the information been collected in other localities and is it reasonable to assume that the same conditions will apply? Gathering data *can* be a delaying tactic to avoid doing something about an obvious problem.[15] For example, surveys have shown that elderly people without cars find it difficult to get to hospitals served by poor public transport. It is reasonable to assume that this applies in most localities with poor public transport. So, only collect information if the answer to a question really is not known. Have the views of the clients been sought? Do they see this as a need?

What are the aims and the appropriate response to the need?

Health promotion cannot solve all problems or meet all health needs. First of all, you need to be clear what the need is, then what your aims are for meeting that need, then what is the appropriate way to meet it.

For example, there may be an identified need to increase the uptake of immunisation. The aim is to achieve an 80 per cent uptake rate and you then need to decide the appropriate way to achieve it. It would be all too easy in this case to say that 'there is a need for a health education campaign to get parents to have their children immunised' because messages about attending immunisation clinics may be seen to be the answer. But this may make no difference because the appropriate response is to educate the health professionals who are found to be withholding immunisation wrongly when a child has only a mild cold, and to move the time and place of the clinics so that working mothers without cars are able to bring their children. (See the section on setting aims and objectives in Chapter 6 on *Planning* for a more detailed discussion of setting aims and objectives and identifying appropriate responses.)

In the following case study, we assess an identified need for health promotion, applying the four assessment questions.

Case study—Assessing health promotion needs

A community clinic[16]

The health visitors and primary care manager in a clinic wanted to make it into a focus for the local community. They felt that the clinic was an underused local asset, and that the health visitors were failing to meet local needs and should extend their client group beyond mothers and babies to include more elderly and middle-aged people, and school-children. They also wanted to extend their role to become health advisers and counsellors.

The health visitors believed that offering an improved service would give them more satisfying jobs. They put considerable time and energy into planning how to achieve these goals. Yet much of the project never got off the ground and in the end the service remained virtually unchanged. Although some reasons for this, such as staff changes, were outside the project's control, lack of clear ideas about how best to achieve the changes they wanted weakened the project from the start.

1. What sort of need is it?

Those involved in the project were anxious not to reinvent the wheel and made a number of contacts with other health visitors who had developed similar

continued on next page

continued

schemes. This is a normative need based on a professional view. It is also a comparative need based on what other clinics provide.

2. Who decided that there is a need?
The professionals (the health visitors) decided the views of existing and potential client groups were not sought. A letter was sent to existing users of the service informing them of the proposed changes. No attempt was made to find out the needs and views of the additional client groups the health visitors wished to serve, although a plan was made to administer a questionnaire (see Question three for the outcome of this).

The other members of the primary health care team were not involved, and the receptionists were unsure about what was being proposed. Neither local community groups nor other local health promoters had been involved in drawing up the plans.

3. What are the grounds for deciding there is a need?
The grounds were the comparative underuse of the clinic, as perceived by the health visitors and primary care manager. The proposed changes were not tied into the major priorities and objectives for the Community Unit, and the manager of the Community Unit and the Unit Management Board were not involved in discussions. As a result a proposal to gather information from users about their need for services which the clinic could provide was the subject of cuts.

4. What are the aims and the appropriate response to the need?
The aims were not clear, and therefore the appropriate response to achieve the aims were not clearly thought through either. One aim seemed to be to make the clinic accessible and attractive to a wider range of groups in the community. Who these potential users were, and what their specific needs were remained unknown.

Another aim seemed to be for the health visitors to spend more time in face-to-face contacts with clients, acting as advisers and counsellors. Drop-in sessions were put on and advertised on a poster at the clinic. These sessions were found to be underused and almost only existing users—mothers and babies—were attending them. This is not surprising when there was so little marketing of the new service. Attempts at proper counselling sessions were often frustrated by the receptionists who continued to put telephone calls through.

Exercise—Assessing a health promotion need

Use the following questions (discussed above in detail) to assess a health promotion need which you have identified in your own work, or one which you are likely to meet.

1. What sort of need is it?
2. Who decided that there is a need?
3. What are the grounds for deciding that there is a need?
4. What are the aims and appropriate response to the need?

Setting Health Promotion Priorities

You may have a huge workload of health promotion needs which you feel should be met, but there are always constraints on time, resources and energy. Spreading efforts a mile wide and an inch deep is probably useless and concentrating effort on priority areas is more effective and rewarding. Before attempting to set priorities it is helpful to analyse current 'real-life' practice and recognise the wide range of criteria which will affect such decisions.

Exercise—Analysing the 'real-life' reasons for health promotion priorities

Identify a health promotion activity which has a high priority in your work; this could be work which you undertake with a number of clients (eg. antenatal education) or just one (eg. a particular patient); it could be part of your usual work or a special event such as a campaign. (It will be especially helpful for the purposes of this exercise if you can identify an area of work which has recently become a priority.)

Now work through the following tasks.

1. Identify who it was who decided that this work should take priority (eg. you? your seniors? your clients? all three?)
2. List ALL THE POSSIBLE REASONS why this work has priority—include the reasons that you are sure about as well as any that are speculation.

   Your reasons could include any of the following, and probably many more:
   - I feel that it's important
   - it is established policy of senior officers
   - we've always done it and saw no reason to change
   - there was pressure from the public
   - it was in response to a crisis
   - we had to be seen to be doing something
   - there is new evidence of need
   - there is evidence that the work has been effective in a similar area
   - someone has a personal enthusiasm for it (a bee in his bonnet)
   - it was the current national/local theme (eg. World AIDS Day)
   - we had a new staff member with special expertise which we wanted to use
   - we had to economise and be more efficient
   - it was politically expedient
3. Identify what you think the most important reasons are. Do you think that they are sound reasons for setting priorities?

There can be no watertight method for setting priorities because priorities ultimately depend upon the value-judgments of the workers involved, but it may be helpful to work through the following checklist.

Exercise—Setting priorities for health promotion

1. Health promotion issues, approaches and activities

Do you define your priorities in terms of:

- issues which have an influence on health (eg. poverty, unemployment, racism, ageism, inequalities)
- health promotion approaches (eg. medical, behaviour change, educational, client-centred, societal/environmental change)
- health promotion activities (preventive health services, community-based work, organisational development, economic and regulatory activities, environmental measures, health education programmes, healthy public policies)
- health problems (eg. heart disease, food poisoning, cancer, HIV/AIDS, overweight, mental health problems)?

Why?

2. Consumer groups

Who are the people your health promotion is aimed at:

- policy makers and planners?
- individual clients or service users?
- families?
- selected groups?
- the whole community? If so, how do you define your 'community'?

Why?

3. Age groups

Do you define your priority consumer groups further in terms of age:

- children, young people, parents, elderly, etc?

Why?

4. 'At-risk' groups

Do you define your priority consumer groups further in terms of high-risk categories, such as smokers, people with high blood pressure, unemployed people or those living on low incomes?

If so, why? Have you examined the evidence leading to the identification of these 'at-risk' groups?

5. Effectiveness

Have you any evidence that health promotion in your priority area is likely to be effective?

6. Feasibility

Is it feasible for you to spend time with your priority groups?

Do you have access to these groups?

Do you have credibility with these groups?

Do you have the skills and resources to work with these groups?

7. Working with other people

Do you know what work is already being done with your priority groups, by other health promoters, community groups and voluntary organisations?

Are you sure that your work will complement any other work which is going on —and not be seen as duplication or interference?

continued on next page

continued

Does your work fit in with existing local strategies and plans for health promotion?

8. Ethics
Are there ethical aspects to your work which you need to consider?
Is your work ethically acceptable to you?
Will it be acceptable to your consumer groups?
Will it be congruent with their values?
How may the desired outcome affect their lives?

9. Add anything else which you feel it is important to consider
Now identify your *top priority* and add any other *high priorities*.

Notes, References and Further Reading

1 See, for example:

Centre for Health Services Studies, University of Kent at Canterbury, in collaboration with Brighton Health Authority, Brighton Borough Council, Hove Borough Council, Lewes District Council, East Sussex County Council (1989) *An Apple a Day . . . ? A Study of Lifestyles and Health in the Brighton Health District*. University of Kent at Canterbury.

This report can be obtained from the Department of Public Health, Brighton Health Authority, Brighton General Hospital, Elm Grove, Brighton BN2 3EW.

Healthy Sheffield 2000 is an interagency initiative involving Sheffield City Council, Sheffield Community Health Council, Sheffield Council for Racial Equality, Sheffield Health Authority, Sheffield Family Health Services Authority, Sheffield Polytechnic and Voluntary Action Sheffield. It is developing and implementing a Public Health Strategy for Sheffield. A report is available:

HS2000 Support Unit (1989) *Health Sheffield 2000—Annual Review 1989*. Sheffield City Council. It can be obtained from the HS2000 Support Unit, 1 Barkers Pool, Sheffield S1 1EN.

The City & Hackney Integrated Planning Group for Public Health and Primary Care, is a new forum for joint working in public health in City & Hackney. It is a joint initiative by the health authority, the local authority, the family health services authority and voluntary agencies. For further information contact:

Department of Public Health, City & Hackney Health Authority, St Leonard's, Nuttall Street, London N1 5LZ, or

Chief Executive & Town Clerk, London Borough of Hackney, The Town Hall, Mare Street, Hackney, London E8 1EA.

2 For further reading on planning, see:

Tones K, Tilford S & Robinson Y (1990) *Health Education: Effectiveness and Efficiency*. London: Chapman & Hall

3 This is a classic analysis of the concept of 'need', based on:

Bradshaw J (1972) The concept of social need. *New Society*, 19 (30 March), 640–643

4 Cooper M (1975) *Rationing Health Care*. London: Croom Helm, p 20

5 See, for example:

Winn E & Quick A (1989) *User-friendly Services—Guidelines for Managers of Community Health Services*. London: King's Fund Centre

6 DHSS (1983) *Management Inquiry Report (The Griffiths Report)* DHSS, p 9

7 For example, Wear Valley District Council have introduced a Wear Fit Campaign, one of whose aims is to increase the range of fitness options available to local people. See:

Simnett I (1991) *Promoting Health—Local Authorities in Action*. London: Health Education Authority

It is important to remember that some groups may need help in order to make choices about what they receive. One way of achieving this is through the use of advocates. See:

Cornwell J & Gordan P (1984) *An Experiment in Advocacy. The Hackney Multi-ethnic Women's Health Project*. London: King's Fund Centre

Braisby D *et al* (1988) *Changing Futures: Housing and Support Services for People Discharged from Psychiatric Hospitals*. London: King Edward's Hospital Fund for London

8 For further reading on marketing, see:

Willsmer L (1976) *The Basic Arts of Marketing*. London: Business Books

Druce R & Carter S (1988) *The Marketing Handbook—a Guide for Voluntary and Non-profit-making Organisations*. Cambridge: National Extension College in association with Channel Four and Yorkshire Television

Cannon T (1986) *Basic Marketing—Principles and Practice*. London: Cassell

For further reading on customer service, see:

Hopson B & Scally M (1989) *12 Steps to Success through Service*. Leeds: Lifeskills Associates

For information on market research studies related to health promotion, see:

Luck M, Lawrence B, Pocock R & Reilly K (1988) *Consumer and Market Research in Health Care*. London: Chapman & Hall

For a discussion on the use of market research in health promotion, see:

Farrell E (1986) *Marketing Research for Health Promotion*. Research Report No. 7. Health Education Council and Bath District Health Authority

9 This is adapted from a definition of marketing in:

Willsmer R L (1976) *The Basic Arts of Marketing*. London: Business Books, p 7

10 This exercise is based on one in:

English National Board (1989) *Health Promotion in Primary Health Care—an Open Learning Package for Practice Nurses*. English National Board with Learning Materials Design, Introduction, p 8. Reproduced by kind permission of the English National Board.

11 Further reading on epidemiology:

Walters W E & Cliff K S (1983) *Community Medicine—A Textbook for Nurses and Health Visitors*. London: Croom Helm

Rose G & Barker D J P (1986) *Epidemiology for the Uninitiated*. London: British Medical Journal

Donaldson R J & Donaldson L J (1983, updated 1988) *Essential Community Medicine*. Lancaster: MTP Press

Alderson M (1988) *Mortality, Morbidity and Health Statistics*. London: Macmillan Press

Jones K & Moon G (1987) *Health, Disease and Society*. London: Routledge & Kegan Paul

Smith A & Jacobson B (eds) (1988) *The Nation's Health: A Strategy for the 1990s*. King Edward's Hospital Fund for London

12 For a critique of the limits and potential of user surveys, see:

Winn E & Quick A (1989) *User-friendly Services—Guidelines for Managers of Community Health Services*. London: King's Fund Centre, Section 6

For critical reviews of surveys in health and health care see:

Cartwright A (1983) *Health Surveys in Practice and in Potential*. King Edward's Hospital Fund for London. (Includes chapters on measures of health and sickness, assessment of needs and methodological issues such as techniques of interviewing and questionnaire design.)

McIver S & Carr-Hill R (1989) *The NHS and its Customers 1*. York University: Centre for Health Economics

For guidance on how to conduct effective surveys, see:

Dixon P & Carr-Hill R (1989) *The NHS and its Customers 2*. York University: Centre for Health Economics

Dixon P & Carr-Hill R (1989) *The NHS and its Customers 3*. York University: Centre for Health Economics

At a more local level, consultants and registrars in public health medicine may know of relevant surveys. Sometimes university departments of community medicine employ research staff who undertake surveys. Community Health Councils also often conduct surveys of patients. It may be useful to ask the CHC who and what has been surveyed in the past, and whether improvements resulted.

13 Maxwell & Weaver identify a spectrum, ranging from consumer protection, through open managerial decision-making, full management participation by public representatives, to heightened individual and communal responsibility and power. See:

Maxwell R & Weaver N (eds) (1984) *Public Participation in Health*. King Edward's Hospital Fund for London

14 See, for example, the *British Medical Journal* series of personal views, some of which portray the experiences of doctors getting a taste of their own medicine:

Britten N (1988) Personal view. *British Medical Journal*, **296**, 1191
Goodman S (1988) Personal view. *British Medical Journal*, **296**, 1396

15 See, for example, a case study described in:

Kalsi N & Constantinides P (1989) *Working Towards Racial Equality—Haringey Experience*. London: King's Fund Primary Health Care Group and Haringey Health Authority

The group concluded that a survey of the needs of elderly people from ethnic minority groups had revealed little that was new but had acted as a very successful delaying tactic.

16 This case study is based on a more detailed one in:

Winn E & Quick A (1989) *User-friendly Services—Guidelines for Managers of Health Services*. London: King's Fund Centre, 22–24.

Chapter 6
Planning and Evaluating

Summary

This chapter identifies a seven-stage planning and evaluation cycle:

(1) identify needs and priorities;
(2) set aims and objectives;
(3) decide the best way of achieving aims;
(4) identify resources;
(5) plan evaluation methods;
(6) set an action plan;
(7) action!

Examples are given of aims and objectives and action plans, and there are exercises on setting aims and objectives and using the planning framework to turn ideas into action.

The Planning and Evaluation Process

Planning is a *process* which ends up with a plan; at its very simplest, a plan should give you the answers to three questions:

- what am I trying to achieve?
- what am I going to do?
- how will I know whether I have been successful?

If you are really clear on these three issues you should be well on the way to effective and efficient health promotion work.

The first question 'what am I trying to achieve?' is concerned with identifying needs and priorities and then being clear about your specific aims and objectives, which we discuss in more detail below.

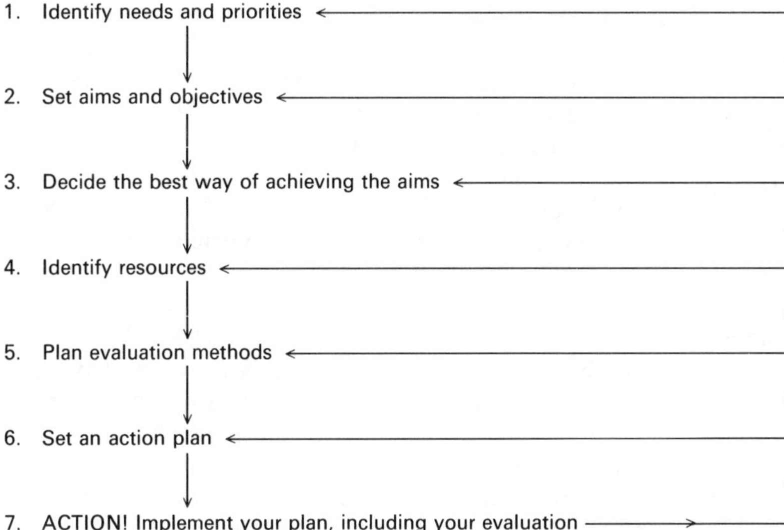
1. Identify needs and priorities
2. Set aims and objectives
3. Decide the best way of achieving the aims
4. Identify resources
5. Plan evaluation methods
6. Set an action plan
7. ACTION! Implement your plan, including your evaluation

Fig. 5 A flowchart for planning and evaluating health promotion.

The second question 'what am I going to do?' can be helpfully broken down into smaller steps:

- selecting the best way of achieving your aims from a variety of possible ways;
- identifying the resources you are going to use;
- setting a clear action plan of who does what and when.

The third question 'how will I know whether I have been successful?' means that you will need to include plans for evaluation in your overall plan. This highlights a very important point: that evaluation is an integral part of your overall plan, not tacked on as an afterthought. It is all too easy to plan a project, carry it out, and *then* think about evaluating it, often too late to capture the information you need.

Putting these together, we have a seven-stage flowchart (Figure 5). There are three key points to note about using the flowchart. One is that the arrows on the flowchart lead you round in a circle. This is because, as you carry out your plan and evaluation, you will probably find things which make you rethink and change your original ideas, for example, working on a client need you found you had overlooked, scaling down your objectives because they were too ambitious, or using different educational or publicity materials because you found that they were not as useful or effective as you had hoped.

The second point is that the main direction of the arrows is in an anti-clockwise direction, but, in reality, planning is not a tidy process. You may actually start at Stage six with a basic idea of something you would like to do. Then you think more about it, and this leads your to clarify exactly what your aims are (Stage two). Next, you might think about what resources you are going to need (Stage four) and realise that you do not have enough time or money to do what you had in mind. So you go back to Stage two and modify your aims. Then you think about the best way of achieving them (Stage three) and work out an action plan (Stage six). After that, you start to think seriously about how you will know whether you are successful (Stage five) and you put your evaluation plans into your action plan (Stage six again). This does not imply that you are muddle-headed or 'doing it wrong'—on the contrary, you are continually reviewing and improving your plan, using the framework appropriately to help you keep on course.

The third point is that planning takes place at many levels. If you are embarking on a major project, you will need to take time to plan it in depth and detail. On the other hand, you may simply be planning a short one-to-one session with a client; in that case you will still need to plan, and to go through all the stages, but it may be a process which takes only a few minutes and does not even get written down.

For example, a chiropodist seeing a patient with a foot-care problem may identify that the patient needs knowledge and skills in cutting toenails correctly. She decides that her aim is to give some basic information and training about this. She will know if she has been successful by getting feedback from the patient about how he managed next time she sees him. She identifies a leaflet that she can give him to reinforce what she says. She decides on an action plan of explanation, demonstration and then getting the patient to practise. She reviews the patient's toenail cutting skills next time she sees him, reinforcing or correcting as necessary. All this planning takes place inside the chiropodists' head, and is an integral part of her everyday professional practice.

We will now look at each stage of the planning and evaluation flowchart.

Stage 1: Identify Needs and Priorities

We discussed this in detail in the previous chapter, so all there is to say now is that you must have a clear view about which needs you are responding to, and what your priorities are.

Stage 2: Set Aims and Objectives

This is the point where you ask yourself 'what exactly am I trying to achieve?' and go on asking it until you have the answer very clearly defined.

People use a range of words to describe 'what I am trying to achieve'—aims, objectives, targets, goals, mission, purpose, achievement, result, product. Although there is no universal agreement about the precise meaning of these words, it can be helpful to think of them as forming a hierarchy (Figure 6). At the top of the hierarchy

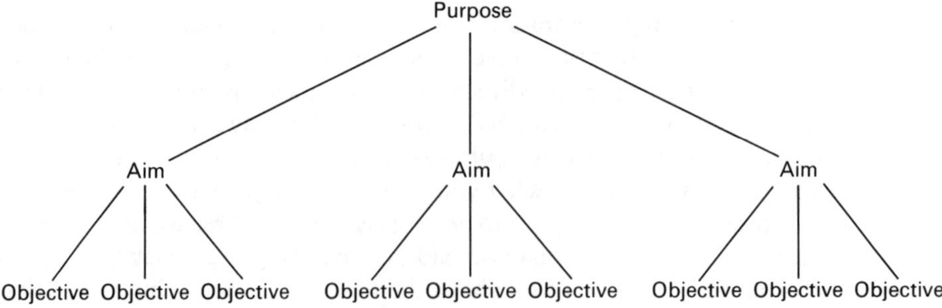

Fig. 6 A hierarchy of aims.

are words that tell why your job exists, such as your job *purpose* or your *mission*. In the middle of the hierarchy are words that describe what you are trying to do in general terms, such as your *goals* or *aims*. At the bottom of the hierarchy are words that describe in specific detail what you are trying to do, such as *targets* or *objectives*.

For example, Mark is a health promoter working for a local authority. His *purpose* is to reduce inequalities in health in the population living and working in the borough. To do this, one of his *aims* is to make health information available to black and other ethnic minority groups. One of his *objectives* which derives from this particular aim is to have a selection of ten health videos in six languages available in 25 shops within four months and to monitor the level of use of the videos.

Exercise—Clarifying your purpose, aims and objectives

1. Thinking of your own job, write down what you believe to be its mission or purpose.
2. Then give an example of one of the health promotion aims you are trying to achieve.
3. Finally, give an example of an objective you are trying to achieve, in fulfilment of the aim you selected.

When planning health promotion initiatives, it is the level of *aims* and *objectives* that we need to focus on. (We choose to use the words aims and objectives in our discussion here, but, as we said above, many other terms are used such as goals and targets.)

Your *aims* (or aim—there does not have to be more than one) are broad statements of what you are trying to achieve. Your *objectives* are much more specific, and setting these is a critical stage in the planning process.

Objectives are the desired end state (or result, or outcome) to be achieved within a specified time period. They are *not* tasks or activities. Objectives have the following additional characteristics:

- *Challenging*. The objective should provide you with a challenge. It should 'stretch' you.
- *Attainable*. On the other hand, it should be both realistic and achievable within the constraints of your situation.
- *As measurable as possible*. You should try to identify your objectives in terms that are as measurable as possible, for example specifying quantity, quality and a time when they will be achieved. For example (using the example above), an objective of 'to have a selection of videos in appropriate languages . . .' has been improved by working out the appropriate number of videos and languages, and then specifying the objective as 'to have ten videos in six languages . . .'.
- It should be consistent with the aims of the organisation and with the overall aims of your job.

It is often difficult to distinguish between *aims* and *objectives* and *action plans*. For example, a dietitian who wants to improve the information she gives to patients may describe her *aim* as 'to produce an information leaflet'—but this is also her objective and her action plan! The answer is to think it through further, and ask '*Why* produce a leaflet? What am I aiming to achieve by producing the leaflet?' It then becomes clearer that the *aim* is to improve patient compliance with dietary treatment, and one of the *objectives* is to improve the patient's understanding of their dietary instructions. The *action* is to produce the leaflet. The importance of actually thinking through your aims and objectives in this way is that it helps you to be absolutely clear about *why* you are doing something, not just *what* you are doing. Failure to think through this stage means that health promoters waste time and energy ploughing ahead with 'a good idea' only to realise, too late, that what they are doing is not actually achieving what they want.

Exercise—Setting aims and objectives

Yewtree Fitness Testing Scheme

The three practices at Yewtree Health Centre have agreed to establish fitness testing clinics, backed up by a display in the shared waiting area, with the aim of reducing the incidence of coronary heart disease in the practice populations.

The detailed objectives are:

1. To raise the users' awareness of the link between inadequate exercise and coronary heart disease, and the part which individuals can play in reducing their own vulnerability to the disease.
2. To assess, and advise about, individuals' physical fitness levels and help them to prepare an appropriate exercise action programme based on those results.
3. To monitor and evaluate, on a continuing basis, the effectiveness of the fitness testing, in respect of the resources involved and the reduction in vulnerability to heart disease.

Ask yourself the following questions:

1. Do the objectives match the characteristics of objectives described above—are they challenging, attainable, as measurable as possible, and relevant?
2. How would you suggest changing the objectives?

Setting Educational Objectives

If your health promotion activity is a health education programme, it is useful to plan in terms of *educational* objectives. Educationalists traditionally often think of *objectives* (sometimes called 'learning outcomes') in terms of what the clients will gain. Furthermore, the objectives are considered to be of three kinds: what the educator would like the clients to *know*, *feel* and *do* as a result of the education (in the language of the educationalist, these are referred to as cognitive, affective and behavioural objectives).

Objectives about 'knowing': these are concerned with giving information, explaining it, ensuring that the client understands it, and thus increasing the client's knowledge. For example, explaining the pros and cons of vaccination to a baby's parents has the objective that they will *know* what the advantages and disadvantages of vaccinations are.

Objectives about 'feeling': these objectives are concerned with attitudes, beliefs, values and opinions. These are complex psychological concepts, but the important feature to note now is that they are all concerned with *how people feel*. Objectives about 'feelings' are about clarifying, forming or changing attitudes, beliefs, values or opinions. In the example above, when a health educator is educating parents about vaccination, in addition to the 'knowledge' objective, there may be an objective about helping anxious parents to *feel* less worried about it.

Objectives about 'doing': these objectives are concerned with a client's skills and actions; for example, teaching a routine of physical exercises, or teaching a diabetic how to give himself an injection, has the objective that clients acquire practical skills and are able to do specific tasks.

In health education, educational objectives are rarely concerned exclusively with knowing, feeling or doing—a mixture is usually required. For example, when advising a mother about feeding her toddler, a health educator probably has several objectives in mind, which she may be planning to achieve within three home visits:

- the objective of ensuring that the mother *knows* which foods are nourishing for her child and which are best given in restricted amounts;
- the objective of changing the mothers erroneous *belief* that sugar is essential to give her child energy, and *relieving her anxiety* that her healthy child's food fads may cause serious ill-health;
- the objective that the mother learns what to *do* at mealtimes when her child has a tantrum over eating his food.

Case studies—Aims and objectives for health promotion projects

Jim is an environmental health officer. His project is to tackle the problem of smoky atmospheres in pubs. This fits in with the overall purpose of his job, which is to work for a health-enhancing environment. Jim works out that his AIM is to work with local publicans to set up smoke-free bars in pubs. He researches the subject in detail, looking at the results achieved from similar projects and working out how much time and money it is likely to take. He then decides that it is reasonable to set his OBJECTIVE as:

- within six months, to have raised awareness of the feasibility and advantages of a smoke-free bar with ten publicans, and worked with at least five to set up smoke-free bars.

Sue is a nurse specialising in coronary care. Her project is to run patient education programmes so that discharged patients know how to look after themselves. This fits in with the overall purpose of her job, which is to care for

continued on next page

continued

patients while they are in hospital, and maximise their chances of a healthy life afterwards.

Sue decides that her AIM is that patients will have participated in a cardiac rehabilitation programme for post-heart-attack patients. Her OBJECTIVES are:

- that every patient, before he leaves hospital, will know what he is advised to do about diet, exercise, smoking and stress control;
- that every patient will be confident and competent to put this advice into practice;
- that every patient, and his carers and relatives, will have had an opportunity to discuss questions and anxieties with a qualified member of the staff.

Sue's programme is a continuous course of group sessions each week, with each session focusing on a specific issue. So each individual session also has a set of objectives. Objectives for the session on 'Eating well when you go home', for example, include:

- patients will understand the basic principles of a healthy diet: low fat, low salt, low sugar and high fibre;
- patients will know which foods they can eat in unlimited amounts, which they should restrict and which they should avoid;
- patients will know what their ideal weight should be;
- patients who are overweight will have devised a personal weight loss plan.

Stage 3: Decide the Best Way of Achieving the Aims

Occasionally, there might be only one possible way of accomplishing your aims and objectives. Usually, however, there will be a range of options. In the first of the examples given above, Jim has a number of options for achieving his objective of raising awareness with publicans of the feasibility and advantages of a smoke-free bar. He could write to the breweries, he could drop leaflets in the pubs, he could lobby consumer groups to take up the cause, he could find out if there are any local meetings of publicans and ask to speak at them, he could conduct a campaign in the local media, he could write to the trade journals which publicans read, or he could try to meet each publican face-to-face. Or he could do two or more of these together.

You are therefore faced with the problem of how to identify the best option. There is no one 'best buy' for health promotion as a whole. Some factors to consider include:

- which methods are the most appropriate and effective for your aims and objectives? (This is explored in more detail below.)
- which methods will be acceptable to the consumers?
- which methods will be easiest?
- which methods are cheapest?
- which methods are the most acceptable to the people involved?
- which methods do you find comfortable to use? (Bear in mind that you may feel uncomfortable with some methods at first, but that this can be overcome with experience to build your confidence.)

AIM	APPROPRIATE METHOD
Health awareness goal Raising awareness, or consciousness, of health issues	Talks Group work Mass media Displays and exhibitions Campaigns
Improving knowledge Providing information	1-to-1 teaching Displays and exhibitions Written materials Mass media Campaigns Group teaching
Self-empowering Improving self-awareness, self-esteem, decision-making	Group work Practising decision-making Values clarification Social skills training Simulation, gaming and role play Assertiveness training Counselling
Changing attitudes and behaviour Changing the lifestyles of individuals	Group work Skills training Self-help groups 1-to-1 instruction Group or individual therapy Written material Advice
Societal/environmental change Changing the physical or social environment	Positive action for under-served groups Lobbying Pressure groups Community development Community-based work Advocacy schemes Environmental measures Planning and policy-making Organisational change Enforcement of laws and regulations

Fig. 7 Aims and methods in health promotion.

Looking at the first of these questions—which methods are most appropriate and effective for your aims—there is an accumulated body of evidence which helps to identify effective methods for particular aims.[1] We know, for example, that mass media advertising is effective for raising awareness but not effective for conveying complex messages, and that working with individuals and small groups is effective for changing attitudes, feelings and behaviour.[2]

The chart above (Figure 7) identifies the range of aims, grouped into categories, and the appropriate and effective methods for achieving them. This provides a general guideline, to which there may be exceptions. (Part Three of this book covers the use of these methods and has to develop the necessary competences.) You may have decided on more than one of these categories of aims. For example, the inputs which contribute towards changing the behaviour of individuals can be complemented by societal changes, so that together they are more effective than either intervention alone (this is known as *synergy*). So, to reduce the consumption of cigarettes, you could provide stop-smoking clinics in combination with the promotion of non-smoking pubs and restaurants and the introduction of no-smoking regulations on local public transport.

The example in Figure 8 shows the range of aims and methods which might be used to promote healthy eating. We do not suggest that all of these would be used by a health promoter at any one time—they are given here to illustrate the range of possibilities.

Stage 4: Identify Resources

What resources are you going to use? You need to clarify what resources are already available (which may be more than you think at first), what you are going to need, and what additional resources you will have to acquire. A number of different kinds of resources can be identified:

You: your experience, knowledge, skills, time, enthusiasm and energy are a vital resource.

People who can help you: it helps to identify all the people with something to offer. This may include colleagues and other people with relevant expertise who can advise and help you to make your plans, clerical and secretarial staff who can help with administration, technicians and artists who can help with exhibitions, displays and teaching/publicity materials.

Your client or client group are another key resource. Clients may have knowledge, skills, enthusiasm, energy and time, which can be used and built upon. In a group, clients can share their knowledge and previous experience and in this way help each other to learn and change. An ex-client can be a very valuable resource, too. For example, a successful slimmer, an ex-smoker or a person who has undergone a particular experience can be a great help to clients who are grappling with similar problems and experiences.

People who influence your client or client group may include clients' relatives, friends, volunteers, patient associations and self-help groups. It may also be possible to harness the help of significant people in the community who are regarded as opinion-leaders or trend-setters; this group might include political figures, religious leaders or pop stars.

Existing policies and plans can be another kind of resource. For example, if you are planning to do work on 'safer sex' to help prevent the spread of HIV, find out if there is already a policy on HIV/AIDS in your health district. If there is, you can use it to back up the work you plan to do.

Existing facilities and services offer another resource. Find out what facilities

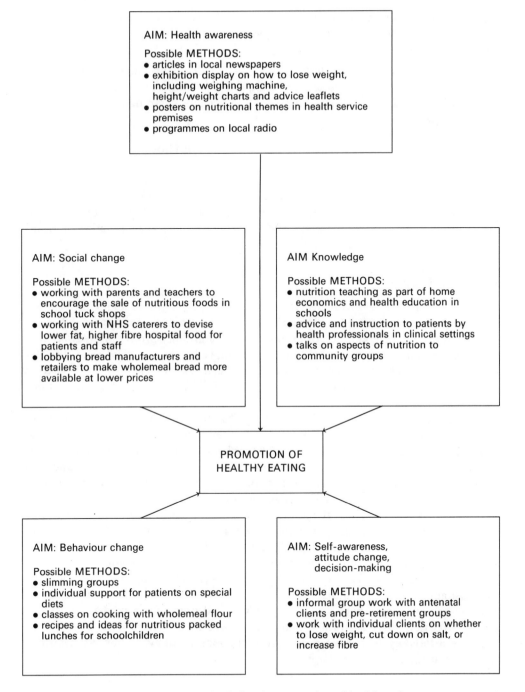

Fig. 8 Aims and methods for the promotion of health eating.

already exist and whether these are fully utilised; for example, sports centres offering facilities for exercise and clinics offering personal health checks.

Material resources might include leaflets, posters, display/publicity materials, or, if you are planning health promotion involving group work, you need resources such as rooms, space, seats, audiovisual equipment and teaching/learning materials.

Stage 5: Plan Evaluation Methods

How will you know whether your health promotion is successful? And how will you measure success?[3] There are no easy answers to these crucial questions about evaluation. On a large scale, sophisticated research is required. This should not deter health promoters; modest methods of evaluating the everyday practice of health promotion can, and should, be used routinely.

Defining Terms

What is meant by 'evaluation'? Simply, making a judgment about the value of something—in our case, about the value of a health promotion activity, whether it is a health education programme, for example, or a community project or an awareness-raising campaign to change local policy. Evaluation is the process of assessing what has been achieved and how it has been achieved. It means looking critically at the activity or programme, working out what was good about it, what was bad about it, and how it could be improved.

The judgment can be about the *outcome* (*what* has been achieved): whether you achieved the objectives which you set. So, for example, it could be about whether people understood the recommended limits for alcohol consumption as a result of your 'sensible drinking' education, whether people in a particular community became more articulate about their health needs as a result of your community development work, or whether you achieved media coverage for your campaign.

Judgment can also be about the *process* (*how* it has been achieved): whether the most appropriate methods were used, whether they were used in the most effective way, and whether they gave value for money. So, for example, it could be about considering whether the video-based discussion you used in your teaching programme was the best teaching method to use, whether the community development approach you chose was the most appropriate one in the circumstances, or whether you would have achieved more public awareness with less money if you had opted for a media 'stunt' with possible free news coverage rather than an expensive advertising and leaflet campaign.

Some other key terms often used in discussions about evaluation are defined in the Notes at the end of this chapter.[4]

Why Evaluate?

You need to be clear about *why* you are evaluating your work, because this will affect the way you do it and the amount of effort you put into it.

Some reasons could be:

- to improve your own practice: next time you do something similar, you will build on your successes and learn from any mistakes;
- to help other people to improve their practice: if you tell people about your experiences, it can help them to improve their practice as well. It is vital to publicise failures as well as successes, to prevent other people reinventing square wheels;
- to justify the use of the resources that went into the work, and to provide evidence to support the case for doing this work in the future;
- to give you the satisfaction of knowing how useful or effective your work has been, in other words, for your own job satisfaction;
- to identify any unplanned or unexpected outcomes that could be important (for example, a campaign to deter young people from taking drugs could have the opposite effect by unwittingly 'glamourising' drug-taking and making it appear to be a commonplace activity).

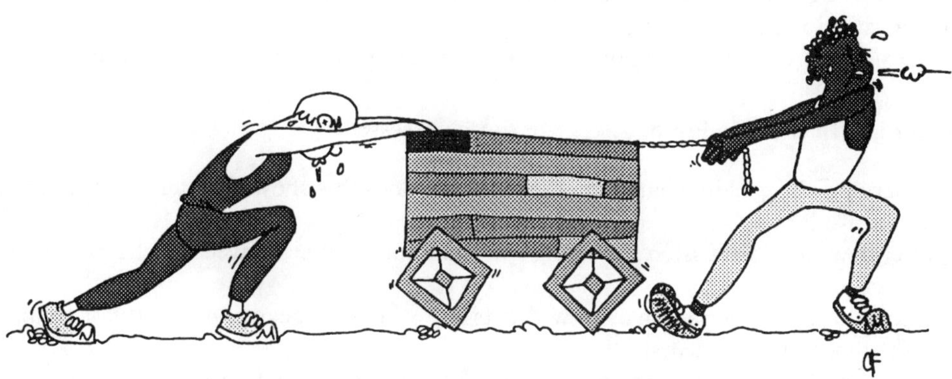

Publicise failures as well as successes, to prevent other people re-inventing square wheels

Who For?

Who will be using your evaluation data? The answer to this affects what questions you ask, how much depth and detail you go into and how you present the information.

If you are assessing how well a health education session went, for your own benefit so you can change it appropriately next time you run a similar session, you will simply make a judgment on how you think it went based on your observation and the learners' reactions, and make a few notes. But if you are writing a report for your manager, or for a body which you want to fund the work, you need to think through what questions those people will expect to be answered, and how much detail they will want.

For example, a group of health visitors evaluating a pilot scheme for a telephone advisory service at evenings and weekends need an evaluation report after six months for their manager who is funding the service. What will the manager need to know? At the very least, she will probably need a clear indication of the use made of the service (who used it? how much? what for?), what the clients gained from it, and how much it cost. It would be helpful for the health visitors to ask their manager at the planning stage of the project what evaluation data will be required so that the appropriate data can be collected.

Assessing the Outcome

Looking first at *outcome* measures, go back to the objectives you set, and plan how you are going to get the answer to the question 'have I achieved these objectives?' Objectives are about *changes* you aim to make: changes in people's knowledge or behaviour, for example, or changes in policies or ways of working. Large, long-term health promotion projects may also have objectives about changes in health status. The following list indicates the kind of changes which may be reflected in your objectives, and what methods you might use to assess or measure those changes.

Changes in health awareness can be assessed by:

- measuring the interest shown by consumers, eg. how many people took up offers of leaflets, how many people enquired about preventive services;
- monitoring changes in demand for health-related services;
- analysis of media coverage;
- questionnaires, interviews, discussion, observation with individuals or groups.

Changes in knowledge or attitude can be assessed by:

- observing changes in what clients say and do: does this show a change in awareness and attitude?;
- interviews and discussion involving question and answer between health promoter and clients;
- discussion and observation on how clients apply knowledge to real-life situations and how they solve problems;
- observing how clients demonstrate their knowledge of newly-acquired skills;
- written tests, or questionnaires which require clients to answer questions about what they know. The results can be compared with those taken before the health promotion activity or from a comparable group that has not received the health promotion programme.

Behaviour change can be assessed by:

- observing what clients do;
- recording behaviour. This could consist of regular recording of numbers attending a health promotion clinic or bringing their children to be vaccinated. It could be a periodical inventory, such as a follow-up questionnaire or interview to check on smoking habits six and twelve months after attending a stop-smoking group. Records of client behaviour can be compared with those of comparable groups in other areas, or with national average figures.

Policy changes can be assessed by:

- policy statements and implementation, such as increased introduction of 'environmentally-friendly' products in everyday use, or healthy eating choices in workplaces and schools;

- legislative changes, such as increased restriction on tobacco advertising;
- changes in the availability of health promoting products, facilities and services, such as low-cost recreational facilities or more health promotion clinics;
- changes in procedures or organisation, such as more time being given to patient education.

Changes to the physical environment can be assessed by:

- measuring changes such as those in levels of pollutants in the air.

Changes in health status can be assessed by:

- keeping records of simple health indicators such as weight, blood pressure, pulse rates on standard exercise, or cholesterol levels;
- health surveys to identify larger-scale changes in health behaviour or self-reported health status;
- analysis of trends in routine health statistics such as infant mortality rates or hospital admission rates.

It will be seen from this list that common methods of assessing outcomes include observation, asking questions, holding discussions and giving questionnaires. Help with these is given in Part Three of this book, and in the suggestions at the end of the chapter.[5]

Assessing the Process

Having looked at assessing the outcome, we now turn to assessing the *process*. This means looking at what went on during the process of implementation, and making judgments about it: was it done as cheaply and quickly as possible? Was the quality as good as you wished? Were the appropriate methods and materials used? You may, for instance, achieve your objectives, but in a very time-consuming, costly or inefficient way, so it is important to evaluate the process as well as identifying whether you have achieved your desired outcome.

How are you going to assess the process? We suggest three key aspects: measuring the input, self-evaluation by asking yourself questions, and getting feedback from other people.

Measuring the input is essential if you are going to make judgments about whether the outcome was worthwhile. You need to record everything that went into your health promotion activity, in terms of time, money and materials. Then you can make an informed judgment about whether the outcome was worth the cost.

Self-evaluation means asking yourself 'What did I do well?', 'What would I like to change?' and 'How could I improve that next time?' All kinds of health promotion can be subjected to this sort of process evaluation, whether it is one-to-one health education with a client, facilitating a self-help group, undertaking community work, developing and implementing policies or lobbying for organisational changes. An important point to note about self-evaluation is the value of *emphasising the positive*. It is all too easy to criticise oneself in a negative, destructive way, which is unhelpful because it erodes confidence. Always look for the positive, identify the things you feel pleased with, and look for constructive ways forward about things which could be improved.

Feedback from other people is another way of evaluating the process. Giving and receiving feedback is an essential skill for every health promoter (see section *Asking questions and getting feedback* in Chapter Eight). Getting feedback from a trusted colleague on your work performance is a valuable form of peer evaluation. Asking for, and getting, feedback from your manager should be part of the regular monitoring of your performance.

Obtaining feedback from clients or users themselves should also be part of assessing the process of every intervention. The important thing is to encourage an atmosphere of openness and honesty, where problems can be confronted without people feeling blamed or judged as bad people. It can be done in many ways; simply observing clients and users accurately is an important tool. Do they look anxious or relaxed? Do they look interested and alert or bored and detached? You can also ask for feedback in various ways—through a suggestions box, through a sensitive and accessible complaints procedure, through noting any spontaneous verbal feedback you receive or through asking questions.

Stage 6: Set an Action Plan

Now that you know:

- what you are trying to achieve and have identified the best way to go about it,
- how to evaluate it,
- what resources you need,

you can get down to planning in detail exactly what you are going to *do*.

This means writing a detailed statement of *who* will do *what*, with *what resources* and *by when*.

It is helpful, especially if you are tackling a large project, to break down your plan into smaller, manageable elements ('bite-sized pieces'). One way of breaking it down is by thinking in terms of *key events*. Draw up a schedule which shows the key events that are planned to happen at particular times. Key events plans specify deadlines that must be met by the people involved and can be useful in formulating health promotion campaigns, for example.

Another way of breaking down a large project is by *milestone* planning. This is different from key events planning: instead of listing events, it lists a series of dates at fixed intervals (the milestones) and shows what should happen by each of them.

Examples—Action plans

A KEY EVENTS plan drawn up by a health visitor who plans to set up a health stall in a local supermarket could look like this:

1. *Discuss with my manager* at October meeting.
2. *Identify support from colleagues* by November.
3. *Approach supermarket manager* (before Christmas rush); agree space and times.
4. *Convene planning group* of colleagues and health promotion officer in January to sort out who will do what and when, evaluation plans and identify resources required.
5. *Set up first stall* in March.

A brief MILESTONE plan for the early stages of setting up a community health project could be like this, in a framework of three monthly 'milestones':

January–March 1990	Steering group agrees job description for community health worker. Job advertised.
By end of June 1990	Interviews; appointment made. Community worker takes up post.
By end of September 1990	Community worker induction programme completed.
By end of December 1990	First progress report to Steering Group.

Stage 7: Action!

This is the stage in which you actually *do* your health promotion, remembering to evaluate the process as you go along.

Exercise—Ideas into action: planning a health promotion project

Work alone or in a small group

Think of an area of health promotion where there is an identified need, and it is within the remit of your job to meet that need. It could be an established area of work such as antenatal education, patient education, teaching food hygiene, or an area of new work you would like to tackle.

Work through the following stages of the planning cycle. Start by writing each of the following headings at the top of a separate large sheet of paper, and then work through them:

1. Aims and objectives

- ask yourself 'What am I trying to achieve?' Identify your broad aim, or aims, then be more specific and identify your objectives.

continued on next page

continued

2. The best way of achieving my aims
- think of all the ways in which you could achieve your aims, and identify the best way.

3. Resources
- identify the resources you already have available, and any extra ones you will need.

4. Evaluation
- ask yourself 'How will I know if I am succeeding?' Identify how you will evaluate both the processes and outcome of your work.

5. Action plan
- identify who will do what, with what resources, and by when.

Be aware that when you are thinking about one section, it may have implications for the others, so you may find yourself going back to modify and refine what you have already written.

To summarise planning:

I once did meet six serving men (or women)
They served me well and true
Their names were what and why and when
And how and where and who!

Notes, References and Further Reading

1 For discussion and information about the evidence for identifying some methods as being more effective for particular aims, see:

Tones K, Tilford S & Robinson Y (1990) *Health Education: Effectiveness and Efficiency*. London: Chapman & Hall
Gatherer A, Parfit J, Porter E & Vessey M (1979) *Is Health Education Effective?* London: Health Education Council
Bell J *et al* (1985) *Annotated Bibliography of Health Education Research Completed in Britain from 1948–1978 and 1979–1983*. Edinburgh: Scottish Health Education Group

2 Tones K, Tilford S & Robinson Y (1990) *Health Education: Effectiveness and Efficiency*. London: Chapman & Hall, Ch 6

3 For further reading on evaluation, see:

Grassle L & Kingsley S (1986) *Measuring Change, Making Changes: an Approach to Evaluation*. National Community Health Resource
Feuerstein M (1986) *Partners in Evaluation: Evaluating Development and Community Programmes with Participants*. London: Macmillan
Patton M (1982) *Practical Evaluation*. London: Sage Publications
Tones K, Tilford S & Robinson Y (1990) *Health Education: Effectiveness and efficiency*. London: Chapman & Hall

Nutbeam D, Smith C & Catford J (1990) Evaluation in health education. A review of progress, possibilities and problems. *Journal of Epidemiology and Community Health*, **44**, 83–89

Examples of evaluated programmes which include useful discussions of the evaluation process are:

Pye M & Kapila M (1990) *AIDS Programme: Evaluation of AIDS Health Promotion Programmes, Concepts and the Cambridge Study*. AIDS Programme Paper Number 7. London: Health Education Authority

Stewart-Brown S L & Prothero D L (1988) Evaluation in community development. *Health Education Journal*, **47**(4)

4 Explanation of terms often used when discussing evaluation:

Evaluation: the process of assessing what has been achieved and how it has been achieved.
Effectiveness: what has been achieved, that is, the outcome.
Efficiency: how the outcome has been achieved, that is, how good (in terms of, for example, value for money or use of time), is the process?
Input: this is everything that goes into a programme or activity, including money, time, staff and materials.
Outcome: this is the end-product of the programme or activity, expressed in appropriate terms of, for example, changes in people's attitudes or knowledge, changes in health policy, changes in the uptake of services, changes in the rate of illness.
Process: what happens between input and outcome.
Impact: this is sometimes used to describe short-term outcomes. For example, the impact of a programme to encourage women to attend for a breast cancer screening test (mammography) might be assessed in terms of how many women attended; the long-term outcome would be a change in the rate of women who died of breast cancer.
Monitoring: this is the process of regularly reviewing achievements and progress towards goals.
Qualitative: this is the term used to describe methods of assessment which describe the outcome in descriptive words rather than numbers. For example, an evaluation report of a screening programme for breast cancer might include users' descriptions of their experiences ('it was very painful', 'it was quick and well-organised', 'it was embarrassing').
Quantitative: this is the term used to describe methods of assessment which are described in terms of numbers. For example, in the breast screening evaluation, there could be an analysis that x number of women attended over y period, with an average through-put time of z minutes and n percentage called back for further tests. Often, both qualitative and quantitative descriptions and methods are used.

5 For further help on research skills and methods, see:

Burnard P & Morrison P (1990) *Nursing Research in Action*. London: Macmillan Education

Bell J (1987) *Doing Your Research Project: a Guide to First Time Researchers in Education and Social Science*. Buckingham: Open University Press

Parry G & Watts F N (eds) (1989) *Behavioural and Mental Health Research: a*

Handbook of Skills and Methods. Lawrence Erlbaum Associates Ltd, Hove, E Sussex

Cartwright A (1983) *Health Surveys in Practice and Potential.* King Edward's Hospital Fund for London

Long A F (1984) *Research into Health and Illness: Issues in Design, Analysis and Practice.* Aldershot: Gower Publishing

Reid N G & Boore J R P (1987) *Research Methods and Statistics in Health Care.* London: Arnold

For a brief practical introduction to questionnaire design, see:

English National Board for Nursing (1990) *Health Promotion with Older People: an Open-learning Package for Practice Nurses.* London: ENB/Learning Materials Design, 127–130.

See also other references at the end of Chapter Five, Note 12.

Chapter 7
Some Key Aspects of Managing Health Promotion

Summary

This chapter begins with a consideration of what 'management' means. It identifies some key aspects of managing health promotion as: working with other people (co-ordination and teamwork, participating in meetings, effective committee work), communicating with colleagues (communication channels, writing reports), managing paperwork (information systems) and managing time (using time logs and diaries, scheduling work). It includes exercises on improving co-ordination and teamwork, conflict resolution styles, how you communicate with colleagues, what information you need to store and analysing your use of time.

It is not easy to define what management is, but in general terms we can say it is about being efficient and effective in your work. *Effectiveness* is the extent to which the results you set out to achieve are actually achieved. *Efficiency* is about how you achieve those results compared with other ways of achieving them.

We have already discussed some important aspects of management, such as setting aims and objectives, setting priorities, planning and evaluating work. A comprehensive introduction to management is beyond the scope of this book, but interested readers are provided with some suggestions for further study.[1]

In this chapter we identify and discuss a number of additional managerial skills you will need to acquire to be effective and efficient as a health promoter. However, it is important to emphasise that possessing these skills will not automatically make you effective and efficient. A number of other factors also influence this, including:

- The people you work with. Your effectiveness and efficiency is limited or enhanced by the competences and motivation of those you work with—receptionists, secretaries and colleagues within and outside your organisation, for example.
- Your organisation. Both the structure and culture of your organisation will influence what you are able to achieve.

- The wider world. The state of the economy, government legislation, the organisation of local government and the impact of social trends are just a few examples of factors in the world outside your organisation which influence how effective you can be.

This book is designed to increase your awareness of these wider influences on your work, as well as to develop your own skills, both of which will help you to improve your competences.

Some key aspects of managing health promotion are discussed below:

- working with other people,
- communicating with colleagues,
- managing paperwork,
- managing time.

Working With Other People: Co-ordination and Teamwork

Health promotion often involves different professions and disciplines working together, including working with colleagues from other departments, and even from different agencies. Therefore it requires good co-ordination and teamwork.

Poor co-ordination can result in dramatic losses in efficiency, and even the total breakdown of programmes; it is especially difficult when big bureaucracies like health authorities and local authorities are working together. There are several ways of co-ordinating, and it is important to use the one best suited to the situation.

Appointing a Co-ordinator

The problem for co-ordinators is that they do not directly manage the people they are trying to co-ordinate and therefore cannot control them in the same way as a manager can; they must convince people that any requests they make are legitimate. Co-ordinators often work at a modest level in a hierarchical organisation: a diabetic nurse trying to co-ordinate the production of a patient-information leaflet, for example, might find that it is difficult to get the commitment of the consultant. The very word 'co-ordinator' may provoke resistance in some people, because they think they will be 'organised' by someone else.

Although resistance to co-ordination cannot be magically spirited away, there are several tactics which can help.

Your reputation. People will find it difficult to turn down any reasonable requests if your work is well known and well thought of locally and you are respected by those who work with you. So any co-ordinator needs to publicise her work and seek to establish a good reputation.

Good relationships. There is no substitute for building and maintaining good relationships, and there is no denying that this requires a lot of continuing effort. It may be tempting to think that this is not 'getting on with the job' but it is an essential investment for every co-ordinator.

Bargaining with individual people or departments may be possible—could you offer something in return for co-operation?

Out-ranking could be used, but only in extreme circumstances. It means getting a senior manager from your hierarchy to request co-operation through the other person's manager. While the other tactics build trust and goodwill, this one endangers it and may give you even more headaches in the future.

Discussion and negotiation with all involved could result in a clarification of responsibilities and more mutual understanding, leading to you being given more legitimate authority by the group. This could mean first discussing the issue with individuals, and later convening a meeting when you have got sufficient commitment to solving the problem.

Policies, Rules and Procedures

Policies are an increasingly important way of co-ordinating health promotion work. This is discussed further in Chapter 13. For routine tasks, rules and set procedures are a way of co-ordinating.

Joint Planning

In this approach the parties involved not only agree objectives but meet regularly to develop and implement a joint plan. This may minimise the need for one individual to be given the job of co-ordinator and prevent the problem of one agency or department being perceived as telling another what to do. However, it can be a major headache to get all the people involved together on a regular basis, and make sure that communications are always clear to those involved.

Joint Working Through Creating Teams

A particular team is given the authority, training, money, staff, premises and equipment to carry out the programme. The team are autonomous and get the satisfaction of 'running their own show'. There is no need for a co-ordinator, since the whole team work together from the same base. Joint working of this kind is not suitable for short-term programmes, but can be excellent for long-term projects such as a community development project.

Creation of Lateral Relations

This type of co-ordination depends on strengthening relationships between individuals in broadly equivalent jobs in different departments or agencies. This can be done by setting up *project teams*, which are dissolved once the particular project is completed. Or it can be done by forming *interdepartmental or multidisciplinary teams*, who are given more authority for making decisions 'at the sharp end', without having to refer them up the different hierarchies. However, these teams are not fully autonomous and this can lead to conflict with the existing vertical lines of command, and works best where there are also good links between the various managers.

Exercise—Improving co-ordination and teamworking

In the health promotion work you do which involves working with other people, can you think of any ways by which you could improve co-ordination and teamworking?

- What steps could you take to enhance the reputation of your health promotion work?
- Who could you build a better relationship with, to improve co-ordination or teamwork?
- What have you got to offer if you are bargaining?
- Can you think of any health promotion activities that you undertake routinely together with other people, which could be more efficient with a set procedure?
- Are there any ways by which you could develop stronger links with other staff at your level in different departments or agencies, to facilitate joint working in health promotion?
- Have you any opportunities for joint objective-setting or joint planning which could help to co-ordinate health promotion in your situation?
- Can you think of anything else? Discuss this with colleagues who are also involved in health promotion.

Characteristics of Successful Teams

There are different sorts of teams—some are competitive, like sports teams, others are associations of people with a common work purpose, for example, a primary health care team. Successful teams have the characteristics listed below.[2] If you have experience of a team which does not seem to be working well, it can be helpful to consider this list together, to identify the roots of the difficulties. (For more discussion about working with people in groups, see Chapter 9.)

- A team consists of a group of identified people.
- The team has a common purpose and shared objectives which are known and agreed by all members.
- Members are selected because they have relevant expertise.
- Members know and agree their own role and know the roles of the other members.
- Members support each other in achieving the common purpose.
- Members trust each other, and communicate with each other in an open, honest way.
- The team has a leader, whose authority is accepted by all members.

Working With Other People: Participating in Meetings

The detailed planning and organisation of meetings is beyond the scope of this book but we offer you some guidance, below, on how to be an effective *participant* at meetings. As a participant there are a number of constructive things you can do:

- Encourage the chair into good practices, for example, ask for clarification on the purpose of the meeting, ask for a summary of what has been agreed at the end.
- Come prepared and arrive on time. Insist on ending on time too!
- Acknowledge the authority of the chair.
- Do not speak for more than two minutes at a time.
- Actively contribute to the meeting—express your views, keep an open mind and listen to other people's opinions.
- Encourage everyone to participate—draw in quieter people by referring to their relevant experience or expertise.
- Only make commitments that you are genuinely able to fulfil, and make sure you do so on time. Say 'no' clearly and non-defensively if you are unable or unwilling to do something.
- Remember that discussion and argument about ideas will help decision-making but personal rivalries will not.

Working With Other People: Effective Committee Work

A committee is a group of people appointed for a specific purpose accountable to a larger group or organisation; examples are the management committee of a voluntary organisation or the health committee of a local authority. There are many common routines and procedures which help to oil the wheels of committees, and it is useful to be familiar with these. The details will vary from committee to committee, although principles remain the same. Some committees start their life with recommendations from a steering group which include proposals for the interim committee rules. These are then approved at the first committee meeting. After review and modification, a set of rules will be agreed which become the accepted rules for the committee.

Officers

The officers are servants of the committee and carry out its instructions. In practice, these are powerful positions which can be abused and a good chair will work for the active involvement of all committee members. Many committees have three key officers—the chair, the secretary and the treasurer. As committees grow, the officers often need help with their work and additional appointments may be necessary, for example, a minutes secretary.

Chair. Much of the work of the chair may be done between meetings, but at the meetings she is most visible, and is responsible for ensuring that the committee successfully completes its tasks. It is vital for the chair to project her voice during meetings, so that all the committee can hear and be involved. Good chairs delegate as much as possible, to ensure active involvement of all members. The chair also has the responsibility of preparing or 'grooming' the next chair and must ensure that opportunities are provided for the vice-chair to develop.

Secretary. The secretary is responsible for all the non-financial papers and reports and for general planning and organisation, often in collaboration with the other officers. She is responsible for seeing that the committee's work is co-ordinated and nothing is forgotten. Typing ability and skill in the use of words are extremely helpful. Good organisation and co-ordination skills are needed.

The secretary is responsible for compiling the *agenda* for the committee meetings. This is a list of things to be done or agreed during the meeting. It will often include standard items such as 'apologies for absence', 'minutes of the previous meeting', 'matters arising from the previous meeting' and 'any other business'. The important point is that the agenda acts as an advance organiser for all those attending the meeting, so that they are able to prepare for it. The members need to receive the agenda in good time before the meeting.

The secretary is also responsible for the final version of the *minutes*, and for agreeing these with the chairperson, even if a minutes secretary takes the notes at the meetings. Minutes are accurate records of the meeting, and should always precisely identify who has responsibility for what action by what date, and when a report back to the committee will be made.

Treasurer. A treasurer will be necessary if the committee is responsible for any financial undertakings. Treasurers are expected to report on the financial position quickly and precisely at any time. This is achieved by recording and summarising every transaction as it happens, so that it is easy to see the current situation. At the end of the financial year all financial transactions are summarised in an annual statement —a clear one-page summary.

Quorum

In the real world it is unlikely that all committee members will be able to attend all meetings. The rules usually state the minimum number of members who must be present for the meeting to be considered representative of members' views and to have the authority to make decisions. This is called a quorum and is usually one-third or one-half of the total voting membership.

Committee Behaviour

Committees tend to be more informal nowadays than they were in the past. Nevertheless, it is good to bear in mind the reasons for various formal behaviours. For example the 'rule' that only one person speaks at a time, and is not interrupted, is meant to ensure a fair hearing for everyone. The chairperson should not allow a vociferous few to dominate the meeting.

The rule of everyone speaking by addressing the meeting through the chairperson helps to prevent a number of sub-discussions developing at the same time. On the other hand, it may seem more natural and helpful to address another committee member directly. Ultimately, it is the job of the chairperson to set the tone which encourages all members to participate whilst keeping the meeting under control.

For further information, including conduct of elections of officers and annual general meetings, see the suggestions for further reading at the end of this chapter.[3]

Understanding Conflict[4]

In itself, conflict is not bad. Conflict is inevitable at times in any group because of differences in needs, objectives or values. The results of conflict will be positive or negative depending on how the group handles it. Handled well, conflict can be a creative source of new ideas and can help a group to change and develop. It can also strengthen the ability of group members to work together. Conflict is badly handled when it is either ignored (burying your head in the sand) so that negative feelings are left to fester, or approached on a win/lose basis (one person only can win, the rest of the group lose).

Exercise—Your conflict resolution style

When confronted with conflict in a group you work in, assess which of these styles you use:

Style	Characteristic Behaviour
Avoidance	Ignores the problem; avoids raising the issue; denies that there is a problem.
Accommodating	Attempts to co-operate with everyone, even at the expense of not meeting personal or team objectives.
Win/lose	Fights to win at any cost, even if it means alienating colleagues or causing the rest of the team to fail in meeting their objectives
Compromising	Suggests a compromise which would meet everyone's basic needs and maintain good relationships
Problem-solving	Openly confronts the problem and encourages everyone to face the disagreements and to express fully their opinions and ideas. Searches for a new solution which meets everyone's needs as fully as possible

Review this chart with other members of groups you work in. Can you think of situations in which these different approaches to conflict resolution were used? Discuss what worked and what did not. What could have been done differently that might have improved the outcome?

Communicating With Colleagues: Analysing your Communication Channels

No matter what your job is in health promotion, your effectiveness depends on your ability to communicate well. This includes not only communicating with members of the public but also with colleagues. A considerable proportion of your time may be taken up by communications with colleagues, including telephone conversations, face-to-face dialogues and written communications. In order to increase your awareness of how you communicate with colleagues, try the following exercise.

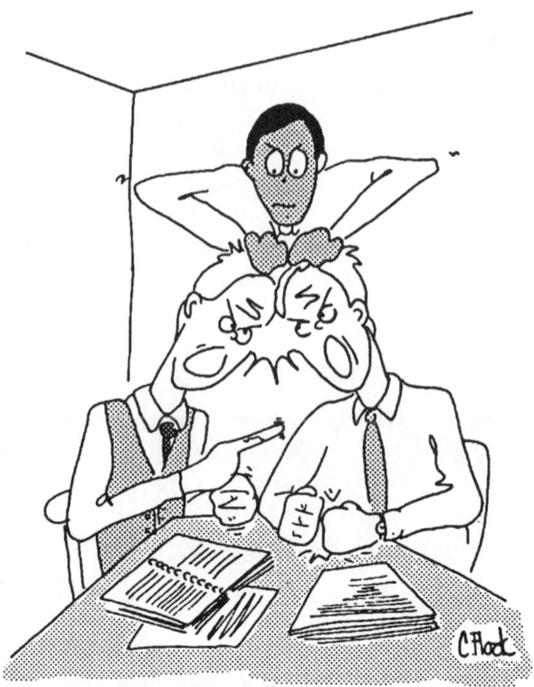

What's your conflict resolution style?

Exercise—How you communicate with colleagues

Record all the types of communication with colleagues that you carry out over one working day, by making a tally of all the occasions in three categories, as set out below. Then add up your total for each category, and your grand total for the day.

You might like to compare your results with those of some colleagues. Think about whether there is anything you would like to change or improve; for example, if you spend a lot of time communicating with colleagues on the telephone, would you benefit by improving your telephone skills?

	Face-to-face verbal	Telephone	Written
TOTALS			

Some fundamentals of good face-to-face communication are dealt with in Chapter Eight. Whilst these are presented with health promoter-client contact in mind, they are also, of course, applicable to contact between health promotion colleagues.

Other ways of communication involve writing and paperwork; these are the subject of the next sections.

Communicating With Colleagues: Writing Reports

An important way of communicating with colleagues is through written reports.[5] With a written message there is no immediate feedback to provide information about whether the message has been understood, so to reduce the danger of being misunderstood good skills in preparing and writing reports are essential.

Work through the following stages each time you prepare and write a report:

Stage 1. Define the purpose —to help to clarify the purpose, complete the following sentence:

'As a result of reading this report, the reader will . . .' What?

The purpose could be to communicate information, to influence decision-making, to initiate a course of action, or to persuade. Whatever it is, keep it clearly in mind throughout all the later stages.

Stage 2. Define the readers —identify the readers and consider them at all stages. Direct the report to the needs and interests of the readers. What do they already know about the subject? How much time do they have for reading? What kind of style is appropriate, for example formal or chatty?

Stage 3. Prepare the structure —decide on the structure of the report. The usual parts of a report are:

- *title*—this should accurately describe what the report is about.
- *origins*—this should tell the reader about the origin of the report, for example, the date, and the author's name, occupation and workbase.
- *distribution list*—it is a great help to readers if they know who else has seen the report. They may detect that someone vital has not received a copy.
- *contents list*—a long report will need a contents list, showing the main sections of the report and the pages on which the reader can find them. This is not necessary for short reports.
- *summary*—this is vital for all except the very shortest of reports (less than a single page). It helps the reader if the summary is easy to find at the *beginning* of the report.
- *introduction*—this sets the context for the report, for example why the work was done.
- *the 'body' of the report*—the writer will need to choose appropriate headings for these

sections and sub-sections of the report. This will be the bulk of the report. Headings should be helpful and specific, and sections logically ordered, with the reader in mind.

- *conclusions*—this summarises the conclusions which can be clearly drawn from the information in the report.
- *recommendations*—these relate to the future, and summarise any changes which the author thinks are needed.
- *references*—putting any references at the end makes the report easier to read.
- *appendices*—a much misused feature of many reports, to be avoided unless really necessary. Ask yourself 'What information will most of my readers need on first reading this report?' If they need this information straight away, put it in the main body of the report.

Stage 4. Write the report —tackle the various sections in the order that makes it easiest. For example, it may be easiest to write the detailed body of the report first, then summarise the information, then discuss the information, then draw your conclusions, then set out your recommendations, then write the summary of the report and, lastly, finish it off with the title, contents list, origin, distribution list and other essential details.

Stage 5. Review and revision —after the report has been typed, review it and revise as necesssary. It is a good idea to show the report to one or two colleagues, preferably those who have good report-writing skills and who will give constructive comments.

Stage 6. Final check —always do a final check for writing and typing errors, spelling mistakes, etc. It can be helpful to ask someone who has not seen the report before to 'proof-read' it, that is, to read it through checking for typing and layout errors.

Hints on How to Write Well

The following hints may help you to write reports, letters and memos in a way which is clear and interesting to the reader. (There is more about writing in the context of producing health education materials in Chapter 14.)

- Be objective—do your conclusions really follow from the data? Have you distinguished between facts and opinions?
- Be clear and concise—for example, use simple words, avoid jargon and long-winded phrases and sentences.
- Develop your own style which should be simple and precise, but also lively and human. The use of active rather than passive verbs will help your writing to be more lively and forceful. For example, write: 'I visited the site of the accident . . .' instead of 'The site of the accident was visited . . .'. It is easier to use active verbs if you write in the first, rather than the third person, so use 'I' and 'we' when describing action. Occasionally it may be necessary to write in the third person, but very often it is not.
- Use punctuation to guide the reader and to avoid ambiguity—if you are doubtful about the basic rules of punctuation, read any good book on English grammar.[6]

Managing Paperwork: Information Systems

It is easy to be swamped by paper, so only keep paperwork that is essential for your job and cannot be kept by someone else or in another system.

Think about who else collects information in your workplace and how they store it. Is there a central filing system? Does it work? Which things could you keep in it? Has a computerised information system been introduced at your workbase? Have you access to it and have you had training in how to use it? Familiarity with what computers can do will not only enhance your career prospects but it can also help with planning your health promotion work. For example, a computer system could be used to collate and analyse any survey work that you may undertake.

Exercise—What information do you need to store?

Make a list of all the types of information you collect at present and analyse it by asking yourself the following questions about each one.

1. Do I need to keep this information?
2. How easy is it for me to find the information when I need it?
3. Could someone else, or another information system, keep the information for me?
4. Who else might need access to this information? How easy would it be for them to find it?
5. How could this information best be stored?

Principles of Effective Information Systems

When reviewing or setting up your information system, it is useful to keep reminding yourself of three basic principles:

- Keep it simple! Systems are only as effective as the people who put in and take out the information. The simpler the system the more likely it is that busy people will use it correctly.
- Do not devise any more systems than are absolutely necessary.
- Organise systems so that anyone who might want to use them can easily understand them.

Managing Time

How well organised and effective are you at your work?[7] The following paragraphs should give you some ideas about how to improve your effectiveness by looking at how you use your time.[8] Time is an expensive resource, and the one that many health promoters find hardest to manage. First of all, you need to know where your time goes, so we look at ways of analysing and improving the use of your time; then we outline an approach to scheduling your work.

Exercise—Analysing and improving your use of time

1. Devise a recording format that suits you, based on the example below.

Then photocopy a supply of the sheets. Use as many sheets as necessary each day. Remember to include any work you do away from your base, for example at home.

If you discover that a particular activity, for example telephone interruptions, is causing you a problem, then make a detailed log of what happens each time. *Do this immediately*—do not leave it till the end of the day. Keep the diary for at least a week. If none of your weeks is 'typical' you will need to keep it for several weeks.

Using codes will save you time. For example, you could use M for meetings, I for interruptions, P for phone calls, IP for phone interruptions.

Time diary

Day ______ **Date** ______ **Page no.** ______

Activity	**Time spent**	**Comments**
______	______	______________________________
______	______	______________________________
______	______	______________________________

2. Now analyse how you used your time.

Each week, analyse your use of time by asking the following questions:

- How did you actually use your time compared with how you planned to use it?
- How much of your time do you spend on different activities? Does this reflect the importance of the different activities? *Important* activities are those that help you to achieve your objectives.
- Which jobs did not get done? Does it matter? Did you finish all the *important* and *urgent* jobs?
- How much time do you lose through interruptions? What sort of interruptions do you get?
- How much of your time is spent on other people's work?
- Do you do the right job at the right time? Most people have a time of day when they work best. Do you use this time for your most important work?

3. Now plan how to improve your time management.

Some of the changes you could make will be obvious. For example:

- You discover that jobs started early in the morning tend to get completed quickly. So you decide in future to do your most important work at this time.
- You discover that you spend about 8 hours each week handling interruptions. You decide to experiment with techniques to cut down this time.
- You discover that urgent jobs are generally done but important long-term projects tend to be neglected. You decide to make realistic plans to ensure that these jobs will be done.
- What else can you do?

Time Logs and Time Diaries

A time log involves keeping a record of how you spend your time at regular intervals, which may be as often as every five or ten minutes. It is very useful if you wish to know exactly how you are using your time on an activity which seems to be taking longer than you think it should. It can then help you to pin-point the source of the problem. But a time log is very time-consuming itself, so is really only worth while if a particular activity is causing you problems.

If you want to know more about how you generally use your time you can keep a time diary. This records how you have spent your time day by day, and you can take a few minutes to fill it in at the end of each day. If you have a short memory you may find it better to fill it in more frequently, say at the end of the morning and the afternoon, or at any other convenient break between blocks of work.

Scheduling Your Work

Health promoters generally find that they want to do far more than their time permits, and that they are faced daily with an almost bottomless pit of requests and demands. This means that, first and foremost, they must be very clear about what their priorities are (see Chapter Five). Secondly, they must be assertive about saying 'no' to requests to take on non-priority tasks. Thirdly, they need to develop skills of organising time to ensure that work which *should* get done actually *does* get done, that is, scheduling work.

Scheduling work into the time available involves three steps:

1. **Identify how long you need to spend on a job**. This depends on:

- *The nature of the activity*; for example, whether it is possible to cut corners without endangering people or the outcomes.
- *How important it is*. If the job is unimportant it does not merit a large investment of your time. Ask yourself 'What am I employed for? Will doing this job contribute to my main aims and objectives?' If not, it is unimportant. If it is important it merits a large investment.

2. **Identify how soon you need to have the job completed**. This depends on:

- *How urgent it is*. Urgent jobs are ones that have imminent deadlines. If an urgent job can be completed quickly, deal with it right away. That means it will not interfere with you getting on with the most *important* jobs.

3. **Plan when the work will be done**. This involves:

- *Breaking the job down into manageable parts*. If the job is big, difficult, or parts of it are boring, try setting aside regular, but small, amounts of time to complete specific bits. Using this 'salami' method (dividing it into thin segments), will help you to see that you are progressing.
- *Estimating how long each part will take to complete*. It can be difficult to estimate how long it will take you to complete a particular task, but an informed guess will at least help you to be more realistic in future! Here are some suggestions which may help:

  —ask someone you know who has experience in doing the job;
  —use your experience from similar jobs;

—consult colleagues;
—build in some contingency time;
—keep a note of how long it actually takes, so that you can make a better estimate next time.

- *Scheduling in your diary or organiser when the work will be done.* You may find that you need to reschedule daily to take account of changing priorities. The important thing is to ensure that the key tasks you have to undertake are scheduled to allow enough time for their completion.

Notes, References and Further Reading

1 For further information on management, see:

Handy C B (1985) *Understanding Organisations*. Harmondsworth: Penguin Business Library

For information on managing people, see:

Irwin R & Wolenik R (1986) *Winning Strategies for Managing People—A Task-Directed Guide*. London: Kogan Page

For help with the management of voluntary organisations, see:

Handy C (1988) *Understanding Voluntary Organisations*. Harmondsworth: Penguin Books

The Open University Business School provides a comprehensive distance learning course in management—*The Effective Manager*. For further details contact The Open University, Open Business School, Walton Hall, Milton Keynes MK7 6AG. Telephone: 0908 274066

The NHS Training Directorate has commissioned a comprehensive open learning programme for health service managers—*Managing Health Services*. This is available through the Open University and locally through some health authorities and colleges. For further information contact The Open University (address above) or The Institute of Health Services Management, 75 Portland Place, London W1N 4AN. Telephone: 071 580 5041

The NHS Training Directorate has also commissioned *Health Pickup*. This is a modular training programme to develop the non-clinical skills of health service professionals including nurses, midwives, health visitors, dietitians, physiotherapists, occupational therapists, speech therapists, clinical psychologists and chiropodists. It includes modules on setting objectives and standards, assessing needs and priorities, managing case-load and time, and effective teamworking, plus modules on Information Management and Technology aimed at a wider range of health service staff. For further information on the availability of Health Pickup, contact the NHSTD, St Bartholomews Court, 18 Christmas Street, Bristol BS1 5BT. Telephone: 0272 291029

2 For further information on groups and teamworking, see:

Douglas T (1983) *Groups: Understanding People Gathered Together*. London: Tavistock Publications. This gives an account of groups, including family groups, friendship groups, teams, committees and therapeutic groups.

For a 'warts and all' account of attempting to teach teamwork to mixed groups of nurses, doctors, therapists, health visitors and social workers, see:

Jones R V H (1986) *Working Together, Learning Together*. Occasional Paper No. 33. London: Royal College of General Practitioners

3 Clarke S (1989) *Seeing It Through: How to be on a Committee*. London: Bedford Square Press
Stratford A (1988) *The Committee Book*. London: Foulsham

4 De Bono E (1986) *Conflicts—a Better Way to Resolve Them*. Harmondsworth: Penguin Books

5 For further information on report writing, see:

Van Embden J & Eastel J (1989) *Short Guide to All Types of Report Writing*. Maidenhead: McGraw-Hill

6 Useful books on writing good plain English are:

Gowers E (1986) *The Complete Plain Words*. London: HMSO
Davies Roberts P (1987) *Plain English—a User's Guide*. Harmondsworth: Penguin Books
Fowler H W & F G (1973) *The King's English*. Oxford: Oxford University Press

For further information on effective speaking, effective writing and reading and effective meetings, see:

Scott W (1984) *The Skills of Communicating*. Aldershot: Gower Publishing, Pts 1, 2 & 3

7 For further reading, see:

National Extension College & Lucas Open Learning (1988) *How to Work Effectively—the Secret of Success in Your Job*. London: Thorsons
Young A (1986) *The Manager's Handbook*. London: Sphere Books
Tschudin V & Schober J (1990) *Managing Yourself*. London: Macmillan Education

For a practical handbook aiming to help people working in the voluntary sector to improve their working effectiveness, see:

Holloway C & Otto S (1985) *Getting Organised*. London: Bedford Square Press

For a handbook on managing designed for both voluntary organisations and community groups, see:

Merritt Adirondack S (1989) *Just About Managing?* London: London Voluntary Service Council

The Open College have designed a series of courses called *Working Effectively*. The courses include: Managing Time, Managing Stress, Making Presentations, Moving into Management—a Course for Women, Interviewing, and Managing Change. For further information contact: The Open College, Third Floor, St James Buildings, Oxford Street, Manchester, M1 6FQ

For further information on managing stress at work, see:

Arroba T & James K (1987) *Pressure at Work: a Survival Guide.* Maidenhead: McGraw Hill

8 See, for example:

Adair J (1988 edition) *The Management of Time.* Harmondsworth: Pan Books
Seiwert L J (1989) *Managing Your Time* London: Kogan Page

PART III

DEVELOPING COMPETENCE IN HEALTH PROMOTION

Introduction

Part III has the purpose of:

- Providing you with guidance on how to assess, develop and improve your core competences in health promotion.

Competences are the combination of knowledge, attitudes and skills needed to perform work of a satisfactory standard in health promotion. As a health promoter, you need competences to plan, evaluate and implement health promotion activities in different settings and with different goals, which we discussed in Part II. You will also need to develop the other core competences of health promotion, which we identify as: communicating and educating, marketing and publicising, facilitating and networking, and influencing policy and practice. These are addressed in this part.

Some chapters of Part III will be more important to some professions or disciplines than others, so you may wish to begin by studying the chapters most relevant to you, rather than going through them in sequence. We have provided cross-referencing to help you to identify which sections of other chapters may also be relevant to your particular needs.

Chapter Eight addresses the fundamentals of communication, including establishing relationships, identifying communication and language barriers, and basic communication skills.

Chapter Nine is about working with clients in groups.

Chapter Ten is about helping people to make health choices, including working towards client empowerment, and strategies for increasing self-awareness, clarifying attitudes and values, and for decision-making.

Chapter 11 outlines the principles of effective teaching and provides guidelines on giving talks, and on patient education.

Chapter 12 is about community-based work in health promotion, including community participation, community development and community health projects.

Chapter Thirteen discusses the politics of influencing policies and practices, how to develop and implement policies, and how to campaign for changes.

Chapter Fourteen is about how to produce and use teaching and learning materials, including displays, audiovisual resources, written materials and statistical information.

Chapter Fifteen discusses how mass media can be used effectively in health promotion, including practical help in working with the local press, radio and television.

Chapter 8
Fundamentals of Communication

Summary

This chapter begins by exploring relationships with clients and identifying communication and language barriers. Discussion on four basic communication skills follows: understanding non-verbal communication, listening, helping people to talk, asking questions and obtained feedback. Exercises are included on overcoming communication barriers and on each basic communication skill.

Good communication between people is fundamental to successful health promotion, whether it happens in the context of a consultation with a patient, a conversation with a colleague or a request to a manager. By 'good communication' we mean clear, unambiguous two-way constructive exchanges, without distortion of the message between when it is given and when it is received.

This chapter discusses some fundamentals of relationships with clients, communication barriers and basic communication skills. The application of these skills often will be in one-to-one situations, although they may apply when working in groups and when teaching as well. These skills will help to develop better communication, but they should not be expected to provide a blueprint for every situation, or a quick and easy route to being a good communicator. They are a start, but improving communication is a lifelong developmental process.[1]

Exploring Relationships with Clients

We begin by asking health promoters to look at some fundamental—and possibly uncomfortable—questions: for example, what is your basic attitude towards the people you work with? Do you accept them on their own terms or do you judge them by your own standards? Do you aim to encourage people to be independent, make their own decisions, take charge of their health, solve their own problems? Or are you actually encouraging dependency, solving their problems for them and thereby decreasing their own ability and confidence to take responsibility for themselves? We suggest that you should work through the following questions, thinking about how you relate to the people you work with.

Accepting or Judging

Accepting people means:

- recognising that people's knowledge and beliefs emerge from their life experience, whereas your own have been modified and extended by professional education and experience;
- understanding *your own* knowledge, beliefs, values and standards;
- understanding your clients' knowledge, beliefs, values and standards from their point of view;
- recognising that you and the people you work with may differ in your knowledge, beliefs, values and standards;
- recognising that these differences do not imply that you, the professional health promoter, are a person of greater worth than your clients.

Judging people means:

- equating people's intrinsic worth with their knowledge, beliefs, values, standards and behaviour: for example, saying of someone who drinks 'people who get drunk are stupid' judges (and condemns) that person, and takes no account of life experience and cultural background—'drunkenness can result in people getting hurt' does not judge the person;
- ranking knowledge and behaviour: for example, 'I'm the expert so I know better than you' is judgmental; 'I know more than you about this particular thing' is not—it is a statement of fact: 'my standards are higher than yours' is judgmental, 'my standards are different from yours' is not.

Autonomy or Dependency?

There are a number of ways in which you can help clients to take more control over their health.

Autonomy can be helped by:

- encouraging people to make their own decisions, and resisting the urge to 'take over' the decision-making;
- encouraging people to think things out for themselves, even if this takes much longer than simply telling them;
- respecting any unusual ideas they may have.

Autonomy can be hindered if:

- you impose your own solution on your clients' problems;
- you tell them what to do because they are taking too long to think it out for themselves;
- you tell them that their ideas are no good and will not work, without giving an adequate explanation or opportunity to try them out.

We suggest that the appropriate aim is to work towards as much autonomy as possibly; by doing this, you are helping people to increase control over their own health, which is a basic aim of health promotion. Obviously, there are times when people are dependent on a health promoter, and rightly so; for example, they may be ill, confused or likely to put themselves or other people in danger. There is also the very real problem that working towards autonomy is time-consuming. However, in the long run it is time that is well spent.

A Partnership or a One-way Process?

Do you think of yourself as working in partnership with people in pursuit of health promotion aims, or do you see health promotion as your sole responsibility, with yourself as the 'expert'?

A partnership means:
- there is an atmosphere of trust and openness between yourself and your clients, so that they are not intimidated;
- you ask people for their views and opinions, which you accept and respect even if you disagree with them;
- you tell people when you learn something from them (eg. 'I never thought of it that way before');
- you use informal, participative methods when you are involved in health education, drawing on the experience and knowledge which clients bring with them;
- you encourage clients to share their knowledge and experience with each other. People do this all the time, of course—for example, knowledge and experience is discussed between patients in a hospital ward and mothers in a baby clinic—but do you deliberately foster and encourage this?

A one-way process means that:
- you do not encourage clients to ask questions and discuss problems;
- you imply that you do not expect to learn anything from your clients (and if you do, you do not say so);
- you do not find out what people already know and have experienced;
- you do not encourage people to learn from each other, only from you;
- you use formal methods when you are undertaking health education, such as lectures, rather than participative methods.

Clients' Feelings—Positive or Negative?

A change in people's health knowledge, attitudes and actions will be helped if they feel good about themselves. It will rarely be helped if they are full of self-doubt, anxiety or guilt.

Clients will feel better about themselves if:
- you praise their progress, achievements, strengths and efforts, however small;
- the consequences of 'unhealthy' behaviour (eg. smoking) are discussed without implying that the behaviour is morally bad;
- time is spent exploring how to overcome difficulties (eg. practical strategies to help a client stop smoking). This will help to minimise feelings of helplessness. (See Chapter Ten *Helping People to Make Health Choices*.)

Clients will feel bad about themselves if:
- you ignore their strengths and concentrate on their weaknesses;
- you ignore or belittle their efforts;
- you attempt to motivate them by raising guilt and anxiety (eg. 'If you don't stop smoking you'll damage your baby' or 'you're killing yourself with what you eat').

To sum up, we suggest that the health promotion aim of enabling people to take control over, and improve, their health is best achieved by working in a non-judgmental partnership. This should seek to build on people's existing knowledge and experience, move them towards autonomy, empower them to take responsibility for their own health and help them to feel positive about themselves.[2]

Communication Barriers

As a health promoter, you may encounter numerous difficulties in communicating. Recognising that communication barriers exist is the necessary first stage before work can begin on tackling the problems. There are no easy solutions, but increased awareness and skill can go a long way towards improvement.

Common communication barriers may be categorised into six groups.

Social and Cultural Gaps

A number of factors can cause gaps, among which are:

- different ethnic background;
- different social class, which may be apparent in dress, language or accent;
- different cultural or religious beliefs, for example, about hygiene, nutrition or contraception;
- different values, reflected in a different emphasis on the importance of health issues;
- different sex, reflected in different approaches, interests or values.

Limited Receptiveness

You may want to communicate, but the reverse is not always true: people may not want to be communicated with. They may be unreceptive for many reasons, including:

- mental handicap or confusion;
- illness, tiredness or pain;
- emotional distress;
- being too busy, distracted or preoccupied;
- not valuing themselves, or not believing that their health is important.

Negative Attitude to the Health Promoter

Some people may be 'anti' you, even before you have met. This may be caused by:

- previous 'bad' experiences;

- lack of trust in 'them'—that is, anyone seen as an authority figure or part of 'the establishment';
- lack of credibility of the health promoter (perhaps you set a poor example of good health yourself);
- perceiving you as a threat, coming to criticise or pass judgment;
- believing that 'I know it all anyway', and you will be 'teaching your grandmother to suck eggs';
- believing that advice will be given which cannot be complied with because of financial or social constraints, or being asked to give up the 'few pleasures in life';
- not wishing to confront unpleasant issues such as the results of medical tests, or the need to change policies and practices.

Limited Understanding and Memory

There may be difficulties because people:

- understand and/or speak little or no English;
- have limited intelligence and/or education, and may be illiterate;
- are being confronted with technical words, jargon or medical terminology which they do not understand;
- have poor or failing memories and cannot remember what was discussed previously.

Insufficient Emphasis by the Health Promoter

Communication may fail because you do not give it sufficient time and attention. The reasons may be:

- it was given a low priority in basic training, so it is given low priority in practice;
- lack of confidence, skills and knowledge which may be the result of inadequate training;
- being too busy with other things, and just unable to find the time;
- managers being unsupportive about time spent on health promotion;
- reluctance to 'demystify' and share professionally-acquired health knowledge.

Exercise—Identifying communication barriers

This exercise can be done alone, but it is best carried out in pairs or small groups so that ideas can be shared.

Consider the six kinds of communication barriers discussed.

1. How many of them can you identify in your own experience?
2. What other communication barriers can you add to this list?
3. What communication barriers cause you the most problems?
4. What suggestions can you make for helping to break down communication barriers? (Share examples from your own experience and make additional suggestions.)

Contradictory Messages

Communication barriers are erected when people get different messages from different people. For example:

- individual health professionals give different advice;
- family, friends or neighbours contradict health promoters;
- 'the experts keep changing their minds' as information is updated.

Overcoming Language Barriers

Language is only one facet of the gulf which may exist between people of different ethnic backgrounds. The root of many communication problems is racism; this is a huge topic, largely outside the scope of this book, but we recommend all health promoters to take time out for racism awareness training, looking at their own attitudes and practices when working with people from different ethnic groups.[3]

However, when we focus solely on the question of language barriers, learning a few key words and phrases may help. Words such as hello, goodbye, hot, cold, food and money may be useful. Help with learning the language may be available from multicultural education centres run by local education authorities.

When faced with a language barrier, there are some useful guidelines which you can follow to help someone with limited English to understand what is being said.[4]

1. Speak clearly and slowly, and resist the temptation to raise your voice in an effort to get through.
2. Repeat a sentence if you have not been understood; repeat it using the *same* words. This gives the listener more time to 'tune in' and understand, whereas if you use different words you are likely to cause more confusion by introducing even more words which are not understood.
3. Keep it simple. Use simple words and sentences. Use active forms of verbs rather than passive forms, so say 'The nurse will see you' rather than 'You will be seen by the nurse'. Do not try to cover too much, and stick to one topic at a time.
4. Say things in a logical sequence: the sequence in which they are going to happen. So say 'Eat first, then take the tablet' rather than 'Take the tablet after you eat'. If the listener does not pick up the word 'after' correctly, he will take the tablet first, because that is the order in which he heard the instruction.
5. Be careful of idioms. Being 'fed up', 'popping out' and 'spending a penny' may be totally incomprehensible.
6. Do not attempt to speak pidgin English. It does not help people to learn correct English, and sounds patronising.
7. Use pictures, mime and simple written instructions which may be read by relatives or friends who understand written English. Be careful of symbols on written material; ticks and crosses, for example, may not convey what you intend.
8. Check to ensure that you have been understood, but avoid asking closed questions that require a one-word answer such as 'Do you understand?' A reply of 'Yes' is no

guarantee that your client really *has* understood. (See the section *Asking questions and getting feedback* later in this chapter.)

Exercise—Overcoming language barriers

The following five extracts come from the district nurse's side of a conversation with a patient whose English is very limited.

'Hello—Oh, we are looking brighter today!'

'Have you been visited by the doctor today yet—did he give you a new prescription?'

'I'll see about your insulin after I've seen how your leg's getting on'.

'The doctor says you should take one of these tablets three times a day . . . I don't think you understand—I'll say that again . . . We want you to take one of these tablets three times a day . . . Oh dear . . . (louder) . . . DOCTOR SAYS YOU TAKE TABLET THREE TIMES A DAY'.

'I'll leave this list of foods for you. There are ticks and crosses on it to show you what you can eat and what you should not eat. Do you understand? Your son can read English, can't he?'

Using the guidelines that have just been described:

- identify what is unhelpful about the way the district nurse speaks to the patient;
- suggest better alternatives.

Non-verbal Communication

Non-verbal communication includes all the ways by which people communicate with each other other than by using words, and is sometimes called body language. The main categories of non-verbal communication are as follows.

Bodily Contact

Bodily contact is people touching each other, how much they touch, and which parts of the body are in contact. Shaking hands, holding hands or putting an arm around someone's shoulders, for example, all convey a meaning from one person to another.

Some health promoters, such as nurses, obviously touch patients frequently in the course of their work, whereas others such as environmental health officers may rarely do so. Touching people is surrounded by 'rules' dictated by cultural expectations and taboos, and by expectations of 'professional distance', which may be barriers to the positive use of touch. For example, a handshake can say 'I'm glad to see you—welcome' and touching a distressed person can say 'I'm here for you'.

Proximity

Proximity is how close people are to each other. Consider the different messages being conveyed to a bedridden patient by someone who talks to him from six feet away at the foot of the bed and someone who comes closer and sits on the bed or a chair. However, people vary in the amount of 'personal space' they need, and may feel uncomfortable when others come too close.

Orientation

How individuals position themselves in relation to other people and objects is known as orientation. A useful example is to consider the messages conveyed by the layout of a room where a small group of people are meeting. Chairs in rows facing one separate chair (perhaps with a table in front of it) imply that one person will dominate and control the meeting, whereas chairs placed in a circle without a table to act as a barrier imply that everyone is encouraged to join in, and that no one individual is expected to dominate.

Level

This refers to differences in height between people. Generally, communication is more comfortable if people are on the same level; so it feels better to bend down or sit down to talk to a child or a person in a wheelchair, for example. Talking to someone on a different level can leave one or both parties feeling disadvantaged, and sometimes this is done deliberately; not offering a chair to someone entering an office conveys a message that the visitor is not welcome to stay.

Posture

Posture is how people stand, sit or lie. For example, are they upright or slouched, arms crossed or not? Posture can convey a message of tension and anxiety, for example, by being hunched up with arms crossed, or one of welcome by being upright with arms outstretched.

Physical Appearance

All kinds of messages may be conveyed by physical appearance, such as a person's social standing, personality, tidy habits or concern with fashion. Physical appearance may be very important to health promoters because of the messages it conveys. A uniform may convey an impression of professional competence, but it may also convey an unwelcome image of authority. Casual dress in a formal committee may convey the impression (perhaps a false one) that the committee's work is not being taken seriously.

Facial Expression

Facial expression can obviously indicate feelings, such as sadness, happiness, anger, surprise or puzzlement.

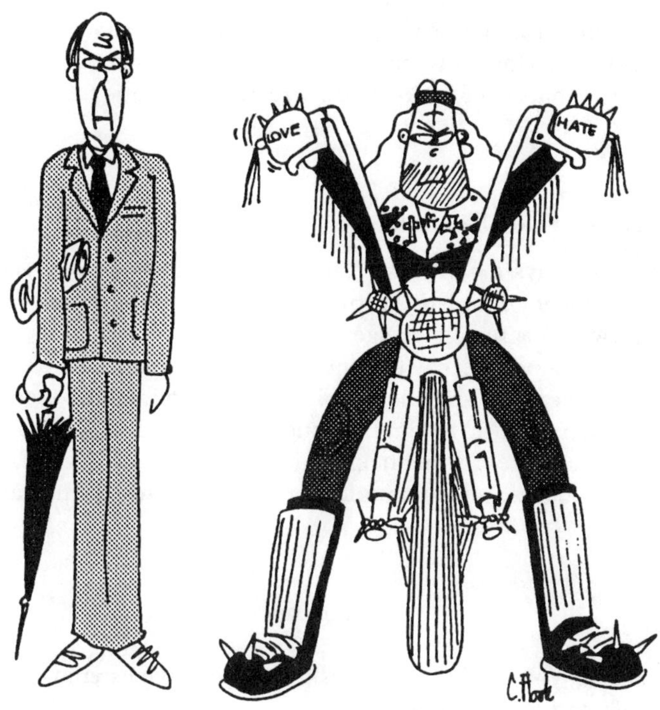

All kinds of messages may be conveyed by physical appearance

Hand Movements and Head Movements

Movements of the hands and head can be very revealing. Nods and shakes of the head obviously convey agreement and disagreement without the need for words. (But beware of the fact that movements of the head may not convey the same meaning in different cultures.) Clenched fists, fidgeting hands (and sometimes tapping feet) reveal stress and tension, whereas still, open hands usually denote a relaxed frame of mind. Mental discomfort, such as confusion or worry, is often shown by putting hands to the head and playing with hair, stroking a beard or rubbing the forehead.

Direction of Gaze and Eye Contact

Whether people are 'looking each other straight in the eye' is significant. As a general rule, a speaker looks away from the listener for most of the time when talking (because she is concentrating on what she is saying), and she looks directly at the listener when she wants a response. For the listener, the general rule is that she will look the speaker straight in the eye while she is paying attention to what the speaker says, but will look elsewhere if her attention has wandered.

This is particularly important if you work with people on a one-to-one basis: a person who is talking to you will infer that you are not listening if you are looking anywhere other than at the speaker. This is most relevant when counselling someone in distress; the counsellor needs to be giving the client full attention, and if the client looks up and sees the counsellor gazing elsewhere, the implication is that the counsellor is not listening.

Non-verbal Aspects of Speech

Consider how many ways a word like 'no' can be said. How it is said can convey meanings such as anger, doubt or surprise. Tone and timing are two non-verbal aspects of speech which convey messages to the listener.

Raised awareness of non-verbal communication can help you to improve communication between yourself and the people you work with. For example, a person who says 'Yes, I understand' in a doubtful tone of voice, with a puzzled frown or with clenched fists clearly requires further help. Words alone are only part of a message, and can be misleading. Non-verbal communication is an area worth further study.[5]

Listening

As a health promoter, you need to develop skills of effective listening, so that you can help people to talk and identify their needs.

Listening is an *active* process. It is not the same as merely hearing words. It involves a conscious effort to listen to words, to the way they are said, to be aware of the feelings shown and of attempts to hide feelings. It means taking note of the non-verbal communication as well as the spoken words. The listener needs to concentrate on giving the speaker full attention, being on the same level as the speaker and adopting a non-threatening posture.

It is easy to allow attention to wander. Some of the things you may find yourself doing instead of listening are planning what to say next, thinking about a similar experience, interrupting, agreeing or disagreeing, judging, blaming or criticising, interpreting what the speaker says, thinking about the next job to be done or just plain day-dreaming.

The task of a listener is to help people to talk about their situation unhurriedly and without interruption, to help them to express their feelings, views and opinions, and to explore their knowledge, values and attitudes. This reinforces the speakers' responsibility for themselves and is essential for helping them towards greater responsibility for their own health choices.

Helping People to Talk

As we have said, the main task of the listener is to help someone to talk. There are several useful techniques, as follows.

Exercise—Non-verbal communication in your work[6]

Work through the following questions and exercises with a partner.

1. When do you touch people at work, if at all?
   What 'rules' govern when it is acceptable/unacceptable to touch them?
   Would people you work with be helped if you touched them more?
2. Carry on a conversation with your partner, first standing too close for comfort, then standing too far away.
   What does it feel like? What is the most comfortable distance?
   What implications does this have for your work?
3. When you talk to an individual in the course of your work, where do you sit or stand in relation to that person? For example, is furniture a barrier between you?
   If you talk to people in groups, how do you seat them?
   Do you think communication could be improved by making changes? If so, what changes?
4. Have a conversation with your partner when one of you is sitting and the other is standing.
   Both describe your feelings.
   Do you ever work with people who are on a physically different level from you? What are the implications?
5. Practise tense and relaxed postures, then welcoming and rejecting postures.
   Which do you normally adopt with people?
6. Identify a few people you work with whom you know fairly well. Think back to your first impressions of these people.
   Do you think that your first impressions were right?
   What were the important features of their appearance which led to your first impressions?
   What is the importance of physical appearance in your health promotion work?
   If you wear a uniform or a white coat, how do you think it affects your relationships?
7. Look around at other people in the room.
   What can you infer from their facial expressions, hand and head movements?
   What is the importance of noticing facial expression, hand and head movement in your job?
8. Hold a conversation with your partner while staring into each other's eyes all the time, and then without looking at each other at all. Describe your feelings.
   Watch two people talking. Do they look directly at each other or do they frequently look away?
   Do they look more at each other when speaking or listening?
   How important is eye contact in your job?
9. Say 'I don't know' in as many ways as possible, trying to convey a different feeling each time, such as despair, confusion and irritation.
   How important is it for you to pick up on non-verbal aspects of speech in your health promotion work?

Exercise—Learning to listen

Work in groups of from three to six people. Appoint someone as a timekeeper.

1. Person A speaks for two minutes, without interruption, on a subject of her choice to do with work (eg. safety in the home, or keeping fit).
   Everyone else in the group listens, without interrupting or taking notes.
2. Person B repeats as much as she can remember, without anyone else interrupting. B may *not*:
   - add anything extra to what A said;
   - give interpretations (eg. 'It's obvious from what she said that . . .');
   - give comments (eg. 'She's just like me . . .').
3. A, and the rest of the group, identify what was inaccurate, forgotten or added.
4. Repeat, with different topics, until everyone has had a turn at being A and B.
5. Discuss the following questions:

   What helped me to listen?
   What helped me to remember?
   What hindered my listening?
   What hindered my remembering?
   What did I learn about myself as a listener?

Giving an Invitation to Talk

To get someone started it may be helpful to give out a specific invitation to talk. Examples are:

'You don't seem to be your usual self today. Is something on your mind?'
'Can we talk some more about that matter you raised briefly at yesterday's meeting?'
'You look worried—are you?'

People who have difficulty in talking about important, perhaps personal, problems may avoid doing so by discussing less important issues. They may be helped by asking specifically 'Is there anything else?' at the end of the conversation.

Giving Attention

This means listening closely to what is being said, and being fully aware of all the channels of communication, including non-verbal behaviour. It requires effort and concentration to listen hard and give full, undivided attention.

Encouraging

This means making the occasional intervention to encourage someone to carry on talking. It tells the speaker that you really *are* listening, and wanting to hear more.

Such interventions include noises like 'mm mm', words such as 'yes . . .' and short phrases such as 'I see . . .' or 'And then . . . ?' or 'Go on . . .'

Another useful intervention is the repetition of a key word which the speaker has just used. For example, if the speaker says 'My work's getting on top of me' you could repeat the word 'work . . . ?'

Paraphrasing

This is responding to the speaker using your own words to state the essence of what the speaker has been saying. Use key words and phrases, for example, 'So you're not sure whether to have the baby vaccinated or not?' or 'So you think some people will be very angry if you ban smoking in the office?'

Reflecting Feelings

This involves mirroring back to the speaker, in verbal statements, the feeling he is communicating. To do this it helps to listen for words about feelings, and to observe body language. Examples are 'You seem pleased' or 'You are obviously upset about this'.

Reflecting Meanings

This means joining feelings and content in one succinct response, to get a reflection of meaning:

'You feel . . . because . . .'
'You are . . . because . . .'
'You're . . . about . . .'

For example:

'You feel pleased about your progress'.
'You're depressed because your children have grown up and left home'.
'You're angry about all the rubbish and dumped cars left lying in this neighbourhood'.

Summing Up

This is a brief restatement of the main content and feelings which have been expressed throughout a conversation. Check back with the speaker to ensure that the statement is accurate: for example, say 'It seems to me that the main things you've been saying are . . . does that cover it?'

Asking Questions and Getting Feedback

Skilful questioning will help people to give clear, full and honest replies. It is useful to distinguish different types of questions.

Exercise—Helping people to talk

Work in pairs.

Each person chooses a topic she feels strongly about (which might be a personal experience or a topic of general concern such as disarmament, going on strike, cuts in the health service or violence on television). Stay with the same topic for all three stages of the exercise.

(The whole exercise takes about 45 minutes.)

Stage 1—Giving attention

One person speaks for two minutes, and the other listens, giving only non-verbal feedback. Then swap roles. After both of you have had your turn, spend 10 minutes discussing these questions:

When you were listening:
- what did you find difficult about listening?
- did your mind wander?
- did you maintain eye contact?
- what did you notice about the speaker's non-verbal communication?

When you were speaking:
- what did the listener do which helped you to talk?
- did the listener do anything which made it difficult for you to talk?

Stage 2—Encouraging

One person speaks for two minutes. The other listens and gives encouraging interventions (such as 'mm mm'), words ('yes . . .') and non-directive comments ('I see . . .') or repeats key words. Then swap roles. Then spend five minutes discussing these questions:

When you were listening:
- what sort of interventions did you make?
- how did you feel about making them?

When you were speaking:
- what interventions did you notice?
- did you find them helpful?

Stage 3—Paraphrasing, reflecting back and summing-up

One person speaks for five minutes and the other listens. The listener makes encouraging interventions as in Stage 2, but *also* paraphrases, reflects feelings and reflects meaning when she feels it is appropriate. At the end, she makes a brief statement summing up the main content and feelings of the speaker, checking with the speaker that her summing-up is accurate. Then exchange roles, followed by 10 minutes discussing these questions:

When you were listening:
- what sort of interventions did you make?
- how did you feel about making them?

When you were speaking:
- what interventions did you notice?
- did you find them helpful?

Types of Questions

Closed questions are questions which require short, factual answers, often of only one word. Examples are:

'What is your name?'
'Is this address correct?'
'Are you able to see me again next Tuesday?'

Closed questions are appropriate when brief, factual information is required. They are *not* appropriate when the aim is to encourage talking at more length. So 'Did you get on OK with your diet last week?' which could be answered by 'yes' or 'no', is not the best way to encourage people to express their experiences of trying to diet for a week. A better question would be 'How did you get on with your diet last week?' This is an *open* question.

Open questions give an opportunity for full answers. Examples are:

'How did you get on at the meeting yesterday?'
'How do you feel about introducing a non-smoking area in the pub?'
'What do you think about trying to do these exercises once a day?'

Note that words like 'how', 'what', 'feel' and 'think' are useful for encouraging a full response.

Biased questions indicate the answer which the questioner wants to hear, or expects to hear. In other words, biased questions (sometimes called 'leading questions') are likely to bias the response by leading the person who answers in a particular direction. Examples are:

'You're feeling better today, aren't you?' (This is biased because it would be easier to answer 'yes' than 'no'.)
'You *have* been doing what we discussed last time, haven't you?'
'Surely you aren't going to do *that*, are you?'

Multiple questions contain more than one question. Multiple questions are likely to confuse, because the listener will not know which question to answer, and probably will not remember all of them. Examples are:

'Is this a serious problem for you—when did it start?'
'Does your store have a policy on promoting healthy foods—do you stock low-alcohol drinks and did you promote displays of low-fat products during the special campaign last September?'
'What are you going to do to get the Council to take all this rubbish away and are you going to set up a bottle bank and get those bins for people to put their bottles and jars into?'
'Are you sure you know what to do or would you like me to explain it again?'

Getting Feedback

After people have been given some information, or have been taught a skill, it is very important to check to make sure that they really *have* understood what was said, and remembered it, or mastered the skill. This is especially important when there is any doubt about how much has been understood, perhaps because, for example, someone is in a state of anxiety or has a limited command of English. There are two key points to note about getting feedback.

It is your responsibility to ensure that the communication has been received and understood. It is *not* the fault of the listener if he tried but did not understand, and he should not be blamed or made to feel small or stupid.

It can be helpful to ask questions in a way which shows that it is your responsibility as a health promoter to 'get it across'. For example, say 'I'd like to make sure I've explained this properly, so could you please tell me what you're going to do about it tomorrow?' or 'May I check to make sure I've covered everything—could you just recap what you understand so far?' Avoid questions such as 'Let's see if you've learnt it yet—could you show me?' or 'I don't think you've totally understood—tell me what you think the main points are'.

Exercise—Asking questions

Work in groups of about 10 people.
Decide on a topic on which it is easy to think of questions—such as pets, holidays, my job, or my family.
Person A volunteers to answer questions.
Person B observes the length of A's response to questions.
Person C observes A's non-verbal behaviour (body language).
Everyone else has the task of asking questions.

Firstly, everyone, in turn, asks a *closed* question on the topic.
Secondly, everyone in turn asks an *open* question on the topic.
Thirdly, everyone asks *biased* questions on the topic.

After these three rounds of questions:
Person A says how she felt about having to answer the three different kinds of questions (eg. clear? muddled? irritated? angry? confused?).
Person B says what she observed about the length of A's responses to the three kinds of questions.
Person C says what she observed about A's non-verbal behaviour when answering the three different kinds of questions.

Discuss the application of what you found out to your work.

Ask open questions. Closed questions such as 'Do you understand?' are not an adequate way of getting feedback. People may answer 'yes' because they are embarrassed, intimidated or afraid of making a fool of themselves by admitting that they do not understand. Or they might just want to draw the conversation to a quick conclusions. Ask open questions, such as 'Could you please tell me what you're going to do . . .'

Notes, References and Further Reading

1 For more on fundamental communication and counselling skills, see:

Evans M & Learmonth A (1990) *Working One-to-One: a Training Course for Health and Related Professionals.* A Vital Communication. Available from: TACADE, 1 Hulme Place, The Crescent, Salford M5 4QA

Burnard P (1989) *Counselling Skills for Health Professionals.* London: Chapman & Hall

Burnard P (1989) *Teaching Interpersonal Skills: a Handbook of Experiential Learning for Health Professionals.* London: Chapman & Hall

Nelson-Jones R (1990) *Human Relationship Skills.* London: Cassell. On building personal relationships; includes exercises for self and group teaching.

Ellis R & McClintock A (1990) *If You Take my Meaning—Theory into Practice in Human Communication.* London: Edward Arnold. Includes chapters on verbal and non-verbal communication, listening, communication in groups and within organisations.

Hargie O, Saunders C & Dickson D (1987) *Social Skills in Interpersonal Communication.* London: Routledge & Kegan Paul. Includes one-to-one and group communication, non-verbal communication, questioning and listening.

Argyle M (1983) *The Psychology of Interpersonal Behaviour.* Harmondsworth: Penguin Books. Includes verbal and non-verbal communication, one-to-one and groups, and professional social skills.

The Health Education Board for Scotland has produced training materials on counselling. For details, see the references 8 at the end of Chapter Ten.

See also Chapter 11 *Teaching and Instructing* which discusses communication and education between health promoters and patients.

2 For a discussion of the concept of self-empowerment, see:

Hopson B & Scally M (1981) *Lifeskills Teaching.* Maidenhead: McGraw-Hill, Ch 3

For a description of the 'self-empowerment model' of health education, see:

Tones K, Tilford S & Robinson Y (1990) *Health Education: Effectiveness and Efficiency.* London: Chapman & Hall, Ch 1

Many of the ideas in this section are adapted from:

Habeshaw T (1983) *Empowering the Learner.* Bristol Polytechnic (unpublished)

3 For more on racism and working with people from different ethnic backgrounds, see:

National Association of Health Authorities (1988) *Action not Words: a Strategy to Improve Health Services for Black and Minority Ethnic Groups*. NAHA, Garth House, 47 Edgbaston Park Road, Birmingham B15 2RS

Mares P, Henley A & Baxter C (1985) *Health Care in Multiracial Britain*. Cambridge: National Extension College

Mares P, Larbie J & Baxter C (1987) *Trainer's Handbook For Multiracial Health Care*. Cambridge: National Extension College

Fuller J H S & Toon P D (1988) *Medical Practice in a Multiracial Society*. London: Heinemann

Shackman J (1987) *The Right to be Understood—a Handbook on Working with Employing and Training Community Interpreters*. Cambridge: National Extension College

4 Material in this section is largely based on:

Henley A (1979) *Asian Patients in Hospital and at Home*. King Edward's Hospital Fund for London, Ch 12. Reproduced by permission of King Edward's Hospital Fund for London.

5 For more on non-verbal communication, see Note 1 above, and:

Argyle M (1975) *Bodily Communication*. London: Routledge & Kegan Paul

Wainwright G R (1985) *Teach Yourself Body Language*. London: Hodder & Stoughton

Morris D (1982) *The Pocket Guide to Manwatching*. London: Triad Grafton

6 Adapted from teaching materials produced by Sue Habeshaw, Bristol Polytechnic. Reproduced by kind permission of Sue Habeshaw.

Chapter 9
Working with Groups

Summary

This chapter is about working with clients in groups. It begins by considering the range of groups in health promotion, appropriate leadership styles, and responsibilities. Some aspects of group behaviour are then discussed, before moving on to the practicalities and skills of setting up a group, getting groups going, discussion skills and dealing with difficulties. The chapter includes exercises on leadership styles and planning a group meeting.

Health promoters work with many different kinds of groups in a variety of settings. We looked at working with groups of *colleagues* in Chapter Seven; in this chapter, we are focusing on the health promoter's work with groups of *clients*, but it is worth saying that many of the skills we discussed in Chapter Seven (such as co-ordination, teamwork, making meetings and committees effective) may also apply when working with clients.

Group work can be seen as part of the movement away from seeing clients as passive recipients of services, towards clients as people actively involved with their own health issues and active within their communities. Many of the groups health promoters are involved with will be pre-existing ones, where members have come together for a common purpose and health issues form part, or the whole, of the agenda. The role of the health promoter may vary widely, from leading a one-off session, to facilitating the development of a new group, or leading a group with a defined life span. Whatever the role, competences in group work are needed, and this chapter sets out some of the basic ones. (We exclude leading *therapeutic* groups from our discussions; therapy requires in-depth professional training in a range of possible approaches, outside the scope of this book.)

Specialist training in group work is recommended to develop skills and confidence further.[1] Group work may only be given a brief introduction in basic professional training courses and in-service professional development; consequently many practitioners report that they feel ill-equipped for the task.[2] For further information, see the suggestions for further reading at the end of the chapter.[3]

First, we discuss the kinds of groups which exist for different purposes.

Kinds of Groups

Groups are not random collections of individuals; group members have a sense of shared identity, common objectives, defined membership criteria and their own particular ways of working.

Groups are formed for a variety of purposes. The term *group work* can be applied to a range of activities from group therapy to social action, self-help and consciousness-raising. We suggest that the main groups in the context of health promotion are formed for one or more of the following purposes.

- For awareness raising—to increase members' interest in, and awareness of, health issues through group discussion. This may be a group already in existence, such as a women's guild, which may agree to discuss a health issue.
- For mutual support—to support members in difficult decision-making, or to help each other to cope with shared problems/disabilities, or to change a health-damaging behaviour. Examples are self-help groups such as patients' associations, tenants' associations and Alcoholics Anonymous.
- For social action—to use the collective power of the group to campaign for social change, for example, on housing standards or community facilities.
- For education—to impart skills, offer information and sometimes to prepare members for specific life events, for example, parenthood.
- For group counselling—to help members to find solutions through exploring a shared problem with a counsellor, for example, a group of menopausal women.

Being clear about the purpose of a group is important; confusion can result if the tasks of a group are changed, especially if this means that individual members have to adopt different roles. For example, an individual will have difficulty if she attends a group to obtain support, and finds the task is changed to campaigning. A new group is required for the new task.

The type of task will determine the most effective size of the group—for example, educational groups may be larger than support groups.

Different kinds of groups may also require the health promoter to take on different roles, and use different skills. *Leading* or *facilitating* groups requires special skills and methods, and the next section is about group leadership.

Group Leadership

Two aspects of group leadership are useful to consider. One is your *leadership style*, and the other is your *responsibilities as a group leader*.

Leadership Style

It is important that all the members of the group are agreed on who is the leader, and support the leader in this role. The leadership style needs to be compatible with the group members, especially if the group has to work together to complete complex tasks. For example, a group of highly-motivated and trained professionals will work best with a leader who encourages participation and shared decision-making. It is essential for leaders to be aware of their own preferred style, and to develop the ability to adjust their style if the needs of the group demand it.

A key dimension of leadership style is where the leader stands on a continuum from authoritarian to participative.

authoritarian | ____________ | participative

An authoritarian style is directive, with the group leader acting as a 'director', who is a source of expertise. If you adopt this approach, you rely on your status, credibility and expertise to ensure acceptance of your views and leadership role. The *strength* of this style is that children and vulnerable people (such as the sick and the handicapped) may feel secure, reassured and protected from harm. The *weaknesses* of this style are that clients may become fearful, anxious and reluctant to take independent action; it does not develop their ability to take responsibility for their own decisions and actions. Furthermore, clients may respond by rebelling and rejecting your guidance.

A participative style involves shifting power from the group leader so that it is shared between the leader and the group members. This means using all the skills and knowledge of the group members as well as the leader, who is more likely to choose the title of 'facilitator'. As a facilitator, you will need to show warmth and empathy, encourage group members to express their feelings, and provide counsel and encouragement. You will need to be tolerant of different viewpoints, showing fairness and impartiality. You will need skills and ability to confront difficult issues and resolve conflict using a problem-solving approach. (See the section in Chapter seven on conflict resolution styles.) The strength of this style is that clients learn to trust their own judgments and at the same time to appreciate other people's rights and opinions. The weaknesses of this style may be that strong feelings are uncovered and distress experienced by the client; this may also be distressing for you as the leader and hard for you to cope with. Also, clients who are used to being told what to do may feel confused and dissatisfied because they are not receiving the advice and direction they want. They will need to have the approach explained to them and be given suitable learning experiences to show them that it works.

There is no 'right' or 'wrong' style and, indeed, most leaders probably operate somewhere between the two extremes, providing some authoritative leadership whilst also encouraging a degree of participation.

It is commonly assumed that groups will be more effective with a participative rather than authoritarian leadership style but research and experience do not always support this conclusion.[4] Rather, we suggest that the reality of leadership is more complex, and that successful group leadership depends on a variety of factors, such as:

- the leader's preferred style of operating and personality. For example, if you have been used to being perceived as the 'expert' with the authority of professional knowledge which you want to pass on, you will probably feel (and look) uncomfortable if you try to switch to a 'facilitator' style without sufficient training, and this will produce tension in the group.

- the group members' preferred style of leadership in the specific circumstances of the group. For example, if group members are low in confidence, they may need you to be more authoritarian to start with, so that they feel secure. You can then gradually encourage participation and adopt a more facilitative style as members learn to trust you and each other, and feel confident enough to join in.
- the group's objectives and tasks. For example, a group which has the objective of learning new skills (such as an exercise class) will need a more authoritarian leader who will tell them how to do the exercises properly, whereas a group of parents in a support group which aims to help them recover from the death of a child will need a facilitator to help members to express and work through their grief.
- the wider environment, such as the culture of the group members, and of the organisations they belong to. For example, the culture of some ethnic minorities may be such that members (especially women) are brought up to be passive, and will not only lack confidence about active participation in groups, but may perceive it as 'wrong'.

You need to consider these factors, and how they may have to be modified in order to achieve the 'best fit'. The easiest thing to modify in the short term may be your own style, but in the long term it may also be possible to make other changes, for example, to develop the group members' confidence so that they are willing to take on more responsibility and participation.

The participative style fits best with the self-empowering, client-centred approach to health promotion, as discussed in Chapter Three. However, many health promoters will have been trained by people operating in an authoritarian style and will have modelled themselves on this experience. If this is true in your case, you will need to learn how to work in a participative style and this could be fundamental to becoming more effective in self-empowering your clients.

Finally, a participative style must be distinguished from a *permissive style*. A permissive style lets clients come to their own conclusions and aims to avoid conflict and keep everyone happy. Helping the clients to enjoy the educational experience is more important to the leader than achieving the goals of the group. Difficulties and conflict are not confronted and the clients may feel neither secure nor cared for. Group leaders may need to build up their own assertiveness skills in order to avoid an overly permissive approach.

Exercise—Looking at your leadership style

The following questions aim to help you to examine your own leadership style. Put a tick in the appropriate box.

continued on next page

continued

	Never	Sometimes	Usually	Always
1. Do your clients say what they feel?	☐	☐	☐	☐
2. Do clients finish what they are saying before you respond?	☐	☐	☐	☐
3. Do you think you are able to see things from your clients' point of view?	☐	☐	☐	☐
4. Do clients disagree with you?	☐	☐	☐	☐
5. Do you explore with your clients the consequences of alternative actions?	☐	☐	☐	☐
6. Do you help clients to discuss painful memories or sensitive issues?	☐	☐	☐	☐
7. Do you share all the information at your disposal?	☐	☐	☐	☐
8. Do you help clients to discover their own strengths?	☐	☐	☐	☐
9. Do you respect your clients' right to reject your advice?	☐	☐	☐	☐

Which leadership style—authoritarian, participative or permissive—do you think you usually use?
What were the influences which led you to develop this style?
Can you identify any advantages in using alternative leadership styles in your work?
Can you identify any aspects of your leadership style that you would like to change?

Leadership Responsibilities

The responsibilities of the group leader will depend on the role she takes; for example, whether she is responsible for the practical organisation such as booking a venue. But whatever her role, her responsibilities will probably include:

- helping members to identify and clarify their interests and needs, and what they would like to gain from the group in the short and long term;
- helping to develop a relaxed atmosphere in which members feel able to be open and trusting with each other, and able to participate freely;
- offering her expertise to the group on the understanding that members are free to accept or reject the offer;
- accepting and valuing all contributions from group members.

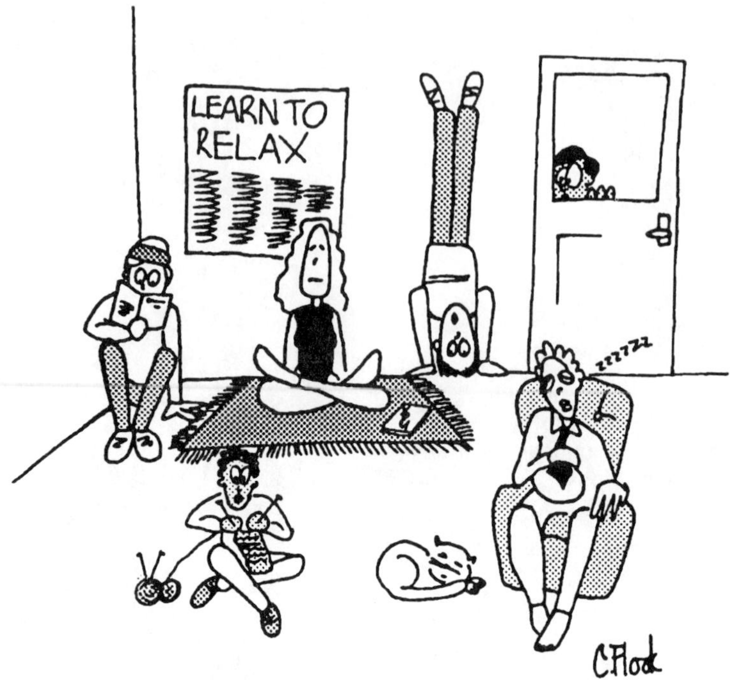

Developing a relaxed atmosphere

But it is not only the group leader who has responsibilities; group *members* have them too. These will probably include:

- participating in the clarification of the aims of the group;
- choosing whether, and how much to participate;
- identifying her own goals and concerns;
- deciding which challenges and risks she is prepared to take: for example, how much is she prepared to expose her own weaknesses and vulnerability to other people in the group?

Group Behaviour

A health promoter will be able to work with a group more effectively if she is aware of the ways in which people are likely to behave when they come together in groups (sometimes called 'group dynamics'). We focus on three aspects of group behaviour which you may find particularly useful: the pattern of behaviour which usually develops in a group's life, the different roles group members may perform, and the concept of 'hidden agendas'.

Group Development

Groups tend to show a particular pattern of behaviour as they mature and develop. This developmental cycle has been categorised as having four stages:[5]

1. **Forming**. The group is in the process of forming. People meet each other, and get to know one another, with each individual establishing her identity and role within the group. The group's purpose and way of working is established.
2. **Storming**. Most groups go through a conflict stage when the leadership and ways in which the group is working are challenged. For example, people may question how things are being done, what the leader's role is and may get into heated discussions with each other. This can be a difficult period for both leader and members, but it is a vital stage in the group's maturing process, rather like the period of rebelling and questioning during adolescence. Successful handling of this period leads to the development of open communication, trust and shared responsibility for achieving the purposes of the group. (See the section *Understanding conflict* in Chapter Seven.)
3. **Norming**. At this stage the group settles down, with the norms and accepted practices of the group established.
4. **Performing**. The group is fully effective at this stage and is able to concentrate on its tasks.

When the developmental process fails in some way, backstage politicking and attempts to sabotage the group may occur. It is thus worth investing time and effort to help new groups to develop successfully.

Group Members' Roles

A study of the characteristics of members of groups concluded that a mix of eight roles are needed for fully effective groups.[6] These roles are:

The Leader. She co-ordinates the efforts of the group and enables it to work effectively.
The Shaper. She is action-orientated and encourages the group to get on with its tasks.
The Plant. She is the creative source of ideas and proposals.
The Monitor/Evaluator. She is good at analysing and criticising.
The Resource Investigator. She has a good network of contacts and liaises with other people and agencies.
The Company Worker. She is good at organising and administration.
The Team Worker. She supports the members of the group and is a good listener.
The Finisher. Her foresight and perseverence ensure that the group completes its tasks.

Each person may play a variety of these roles in a group and most people have their preferred roles. If one or more of these roles is lacking, a member or leader can help to make a group more successful by consciously adopting a new role herself, or helping someone else to do so.

Hidden Agendas

People will have their own individual reasons for joining a group, which may be in addition to, or instead of, the reason expected. For example, a woman may attend a women's health group because she is lonely and sees the group as way of meeting people; she has not joined because she is particularly interested in health issues. Or a group member may seek a prominent position in a group, such as being the chairperson or secretary, to fulfil her need to be valued and useful; she may or may not also be committed to the work itself and the aims of the group. In these examples, fulfilling these personal objectives are 'hidden agendas'.

Most people bring their own 'hidden agendas' to groups, in addition to the agreed group objectives; these commonly include meeting the need for social contact, or making a particular alliance. Members will work together best when there is communication about individual objectives and agreement about shared objectives. Otherwise members may promote their own interests at the expense of the group's. A group leader will be more effective if she is aware of the hidden agendas in the group and can find ways of dealing with them.

Setting Up a Group

Planning and preparation are essential for successful group work. The checklist below takes you step-by-step through the thinking and planning you need to do when setting up a group.[7] (See also Chapter Six *Planning and Evaluating*.)

Why are you Proposing to Run the Group?

- Are you reacting to a demand from clients, other professionals, a community or your own observations?
- Are you trying to develop your health promotion role and see this group as a way of progressing?
- Are you aiming to provide advice and support, or to supply information, or to help people to change health-related behaviour?
- Are you aiming to satisfy your own needs or your clients' needs? (Your reasons can include both, but it is helpful to distinguish between them.)

Who Will the Members Be?

- Will the members be referred to the group (from their GP, for example), will they be coerced into joining or will membership be entirely voluntary?
- How will you identify the potential members of your group—from individuals requesting a group, from local or national registers, from people with shared characteristics (age, sex, lifestyle, culture, job, health risks, etc.), or by other means?
- How will you recruit your members? Do you need to advertise?
- How many members do you aim to have? What is the ideal number, bearing in mind the purpose of the group and any constraints imposed by your location?

What are the Group's Aims and Objectives?

- Are these within the realistic abilities of yourself and the members?
- Can all the potential membership understand them?

- Are you clear about your own objectives in setting up the group, and whether these are different from the members' objectives?
- Is each member clear about her individual objectives, ie. the specific outcomes she hopes to achieve through attending the group?

Where will the Group be Held?

- Is the location appropriate? For example, a health centre or hospital may appear clinical and cold and remind people of illness. 'Neutral' territory, such as a room in a pub or community centre, or in someone's house, may be more relaxing and inviting.
- What is the seating like? If you are aiming for participative group work, seating people in a circle is best, with physical barriers to communication such as tables or desks removed. Can you put chairs in a circle, where all group members can see each other?

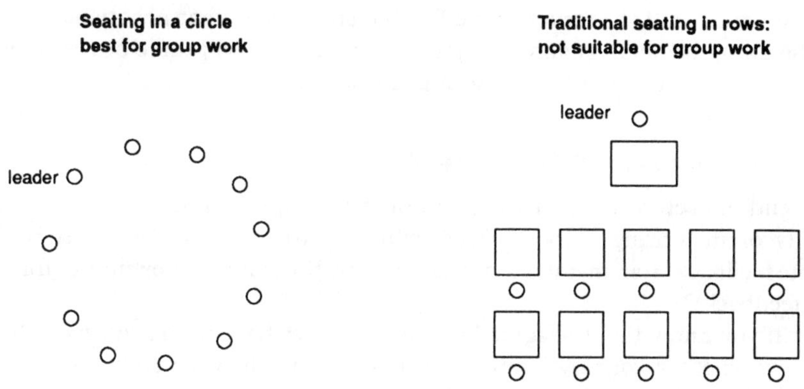

Fig. 9 Seating for group work.

- What are the facilities like? Is there enough space for the activities you plan? Is the floor covering suitable for the purpose? Is the temperature suitable, and adjustable if necessary? Are the facilities adequate for the purpose (for example, access for the disabled, access for pushchairs, toilets, catering facilities, washing/shower rooms, crèche)?
- Is there good access? Is the venue accessible by local transport? Do you have transport for members who cannot manage on public transport? Are parking arrangements satisfactory?
- What are the security arrangements? Where are the fire extinguishers and what is the fire drill? In case of an emergency, who do you contact? Do you need insurance cover?

What Resources do you Need?

- Do you need any special equipment, for example, video equipment, power points? Are you familiar with the equipment and confident you can operate it? Does the equipment have to be booked in advance and if so, are you familiar with the booking system?
- Do you need any additional resources, for example, videos, leaflets, posters, books, outside speakers? If so, have you made all the necessary arrangements in advance?
- Do you need money to pay for anything? If so, have you identified a source of funding (for example, a charge to the group members, a trust fund or a sponsor)?

When will the Group be Held?

- Is the time you have chosen the best one for the clients, or have you chosen it to suit yourself? Does the length of meetings suit members and take into account the other commitments of members? Have you consulted potential members about timing and tried to satisfy the majority?

How will the Group be Run?

- Will it be a self-help group and directed by the members, or leader-led?
- To what extent will the structure be flexible and the content negotiable?
- Will the group be open (anyone can join at any time) or will there be restrictions on admitting new members once the group has started?

How will the Group be Evaluated?

- At the end of each meeting? At the end of the group? Or both?
- Verbally or in writing or both? How will you ask questions in order to obtain accurate feedback from members (for example by providing opportunities for anonymous feedback)?
- How will you know that the agreed group objectives have been achieved? How will you know whether your own objectives have been achieved? How will you know whether each individual has achieved her objectives?
- Were there any unplanned outcomes of the group? Were these desirable or undesirable and what caused them?
- What have you learned? What would you do differently next time?

Getting Groups Going

Almost everyone feels nervous about going to a group meeting for the first time, especially if knowing anyone else there is unlikely. The initial task for the group leader is to 'break the ice' and help people to feel at ease.

On Arrival

It helps if clients can be greeted personally and introduced to other people—giving people something to do also helps: 'Help yourself to a cup of tea!', 'There are some books and leaflets on the table if you'd like to look at them till everyone has arrived'.

Getting to Know Each Other

Knowing each person's name and something about him is the first step towards constructive groupwork because it helps him to feel valued as a member of the group, and is the beginning of openness and trust between members.

There are many ways of going about this, some of which are as follows:[8]

Introduction in pairs. Ask each person to sit next to someone he has not met before —one person in each pair then 'interviews' his partner. After a few minutes (the leader keeps the time) the partners swap roles and the other person is interviewed. Then, in turn, each member of the group introduces his partner by name and says something about him. You may like to remind people that no-one has to answer any questions if he does not wish to.

The leader could also suggest appropriate questions: in a parentcraft session, that partners find out if this is the first baby, where the mother goes for antenatal checkups, or where she is booked to have her baby; in a slimming group, that people find out what diets their partners have tried.

Name games. Group members sit in a circle and you, the leader, take an object, such as a pen, and hand it to the person on your left, saying 'My name is A and this is a pen'. You ask the person who now holds the pen to say 'My name is B and A says that this is a pen'. B then passes the pen to the person on his left, who says 'My name is C and B says that A says that this is a pen'. This continues until the pen gets back to the beginning. If a group member forgets someone's name, the rest of the group can prompt him. This helps to establish a co-operative and supportive atmosphere as well as helping people to learn each other's names. Any tension and embarrassment are relieved by laughing and ice is effectively broken.

At subsequent group meetings, it is often helpful to do a quick round of names at the beginning, eg. 'Who would like to have a shot at naming every member of the group?' or 'I'm going to try to see if I can remember everyone's name'.

You may like to set the tone by suggesting how people are addressed, by first names or more formally by Mr, Mrs etc. The important thing is to encourage people to use whatever feels comfortable. 'My name is Ann Jones, and I'm happy for you to call me Ann if you like'.

Sharing initial feelings and expectations. People may be helped to relax if they know that others also feel nervous or shy. So ask 'What did you feel about coming here today? Did anyone feel nervous? Did anyone almost *not* come?'—this can open the way for people to express their anxieties. You can also encourage them to say why they have come to the meeting and what they expect to gain from it. It might help to ask members to complete a checklist, ticking statements that are true for them. Such statements could include:[9]

- I'm afraid I won't have anything to say

- I'm afraid I'll talk too much
- I'm worried I'll make a fool of myself
- I'll be too embarrassed to join in
- I'm afraid I might get upset
- I'm afraid I may be bored
- I want to meet other people in the same boat
- I enjoy talking to others
- I enjoy a good argument
- I want to get out of the house
- I want to go somewhere different
- I enjoy listening to other people

Each person can then compare his list with those of one or two other people in the group, and it may be helpful to share what has been discovered with the whole group.

Setting Ground Rules

People joining a group will have different expectations and assumptions about how the group will run. Problems may arise if these are not brought out in the open and clarified at the beginning. For example, people may assume that what they say in a group will be treated confidentially, then be upset if they find that another member did not realise this and had discussed the issue elsewhere. Or some members may expect the group leader to take all the responsibility for organising the group, and feel let down if they later discover that the leader expects *them* to do some of the work.

To prevent these difficulties, it is often helpful to establish a clear 'contract' or 'set of ground rules'. So, early on in the life of a group members need the opportunity to explore their expectations, and reach agreement, about issues such as:

- How members are expected to behave in the group. For example, is smoking allowed?
- Are any rules and sanctions to be set, for example, about non-attendance at group meetings or whether members can join in if they arrive late?
- What is confidential to the group?
- Can new members join at any time? Or is the group closed to new membership?
- How will the leader and the members exercise control in the group?
- Who has responsibility for the practical aspects of running the group, such as bringing the refreshments along or booking the room?

For example, in a self-help group, mutual rights and responsibilities will be agreed on the basis of equality of leader and clients. In reality, the power balance will not be completely equal and a contract will help with power sharing. In a counselling group the power of the counsellor is much greater than that of the clients and the leader has a duty to respect the members and to promote their autonomy.

Discussion Skills

It is a fallacy to believe that leading a discussion will just happen by putting a group of people together and saying 'Let's discuss . . .'. Discussion needs planning and preparation, and there are many ways of triggering it off and providing structures which will help everyone to participate. Some of these are as follows.

Trigger Materials

Discussion can be triggered by providing a focus, preferably a controversial one. This can simply be a question ('What do you think about the decision to close the cottage hospital?'), or it might be a leaflet, a poster, a short film or videotape, or an item in a newspaper or magazine ('What do you think the makers of this cigarette are trying to convey in this advertisement?'). Choose something that people are likely to have strong views about.

Some health promotion videos are specially made as trigger materials, presenting situations for people to talk about. Helpful notes for group leaders often accompany such videos.

Brainstorms

This is a useful way to open up a subject and collect everyone's ideas. Ask an open question to which there is no single right answer ('Why do people drink?', 'What do you feel you need to know before your baby is born?'). Accept every suggestion, without comment or criticism, and write them down in a list on a flipchart or blackboard. Ask the group not to start discussing the ideas until everybody has finished. You can make your own suggestions and write them down along with everyone else's.

In this way all members' contributions are equally valued, and everyone has a chance to participate. Encourage shy members by asking 'Anything else?' and allowing silent pauses while people think.

Then you can set the group to work by asking them to put the ideas into categories, and to identify the key features of each category. For example, people might categorise reasons for drinking into a 'constructive' category ('It helps me to socialise', 'It helps me to relax, to feel good') and an 'escape' category ('I can forget my problems', 'It stops me from feeling upset').

Rounds

A 'round' is a way of giving everyone an equal chance to participate. You invite each group member, in turn round the circle, to make a brief statement. You may like to start the round yourself or to join in when your turn comes in the circle. For example, ask everyone to make a brief statement about one of the following:

'My first feelings when I knew I was pregnant were . . .'
'What I think about jogging is . . .'
'The main reason why I can't lose weight is . . .'
'The thing which has helped me most is . . .'

There are three essential rules for successful rounds, which must be explained, and gently enforced if necessary. These are:

- no interruptions until each person has finished his statement;
- no comments on anybody's contribution until the full round is completed (ie. no discussion, praise, interpretation, criticism or I-think-that-too type of remark);
- anyone can choose not to participate. Give permission, clearly and emphatically, that anyone who does not want to make a statement can just say 'pass'. This is very important for reinforcing the principle of voluntary participation.

Rounds are also useful ways of beginning and ending sessions. For example:

'One thing I've put into practice since last week is . . .'
'The main thing I've got from today's session is . . .'
'One thing I'm going to find out by next time we meet is . . .'

It's also a useful way of getting feedback. For example:

'One thing I really liked about today's session was . . .'
'One thing I didn't like about today's session was . . .'
'One thing I wish we'd done is . . .'

Buzz Groups

Buzz groups are small groups of two to six people who discuss questions or topics for short periods, usually about ten minutes. It is especially useful for large groups to be divided up in this way, as it gives everyone more chance to talk. Divide the groups first of all, and then say what you would like each one to do ('Make a list of the times when you want a cigarette' or 'Talk about the things which you find helpful when you feel stressed'), and how long they have in which to do it. If you want people to share ideas with the rest of the group as a whole afterwards, it may be helpful to provide large sheets of paper and felt-tip pens, so that 'posters' can be put up for everyone to see and discuss.

Safe Revelations

Sometimes people may hesitate or refuse to say what they really feel for fear of looking silly, being embarrassed or getting upset. One way of overcoming this is to give each person a piece of paper and ask him to write down (for example) what his biggest worry is, or what he really wants to know. All the papers are then folded and put in a receptacle such as a waste-paper basket or a shopping bag. Each person in turn picks out one piece of paper and reads aloud what it says. Tell people not to say if they happen to pick out their own piece of paper, and that, of course, nobody needs to identify himself as the author of any of the statements.

The aim is to find out the concerns of the group members in the security of anonymity. Make sure that everyone listens and does not comment until all the papers have been read out. Then you can discuss what was discovered.

Exercise—Planning a group meeting

1. Identify a health promotion opportunity that you have encountered or are likely to encounter, where informal group work would be appropriate.

   (For example, this could be a group of food handlers, a preretirement group, an antenatal group, a group of patients in hospital recovering from a heart attack, a stop-smoking group or a slimming group.)

   Assume that your group consists of about 12 people who do not know each other, and that this is the first of several meetings.
2. What do you think would be the best place, time and physical features of the meeting room?
3. What are you aims for the first meeting?
4. What are your objectives for your group members for the first meeting?

   Complete the following:
   At the end of the first meeting, each group member will
   1. ......
   2. ......
   3. ......
   etc ......
5. Make a plan for what you will do
   - as people start to arrive
   - to get people to know each other
   - in the main part of the group meeting
   - to round off the meeting at the end
   - to evaluate whether you have achieved the objectives you set in (4) above.

Dealing with Difficulties

Group workers often find the prospect of group work daunting, and anticipate being unable to cope with problems. A way forward is to acknowledge and face these fears, and work out strategies of coping should problems actually arise. Some common fears and possible strategies for coping are as follows.

Silence

Are you afraid that you may be left with your group in an awful silence? If so, remember that silence can be useful; it can be time which group members need to think. Silence often does not feel as threatening to group members as it may do to you. However, you may find it helpful to:

- run a group with a partner, so that you can help each other out if either of you gets stuck;
- ensure thorough preparation, so that you have planned activities and questions. Write down a plan, and a list of questions to ask (eg. at the end of a trigger film) and don't be afraid to refer to it in front of the group.

- have a 'spare' activity ready to use if the reason for the discussion 'drying up' is that what you have planned does not seem to be working.

Disasters

Unexpected 'disasters' include such things as getting lost and arriving late, or finding that too few, or too many people have turned up. There is no blueprint strategy to cope with the unexpected, but it will help if you acknowledge what has happened and share it with your group ('I'm delighted that so many of you have come along, but I wasn't expecting such a crowd, so we may be a bit squashed this week'). Also share your plans for dealing with the 'disaster' ('I'm going to try to get a bigger room next time' . . . 'I'm going to start ten minutes late'). Sharing the problem and enlisting co-operation can have the positive benefit of encouraging mutual support; *not* sharing it can leave your group feeling angry.

Distractions

Distractions can take many forms: noises outside the room (eg. road works), noises inside the room (eg. crying babies, coughing), people coming in late or leaving early, interruptions. Distractions can also be caused by group members themselves, for example, by becoming very angry or upset.

As a rule, there are three choices for you as group leader:

- ignore them. This is seldom a good idea, as it leaves people wondering if you are going to do anything, and this in itself is a distraction.
- acknowledge and accept them. This is generally best with things you cannot change ('I know the traffic is really noisy, but there's nothing we can do about it, so I think we'll just have to put up with it').
- do something about them, preferably involving the group in the decision ('As so many of you found it difficult to get here by 2 pm, shall we start at 2.15 next week?' 'Do you think it would be helpful if you took it in turns to look after the babies in the next room?').

If someone is showing emotion, such as crying, acknowledge it ('I can see that you're upset'), offer reassurance that it is OK to show emotion ('there's no need to be embarrassed . . . we don't mind if you cry . . .'), and offer the opportunity to talk about it ('Would you like to tell us what is upsetting you?') or to take some time away from the group, accompanied by you or someone else ('Shall we go outside for a few minutes?'). Do not put any pressure on the person; help him to do what he wants to do, whether it is talking, keeping silent, staying, leaving or being by himself. But do not ignore a show of emotion; ignoring it will only cause tension and embarrassment.

Difficult Behaviour

How group members behave can pose difficulties for the leader. There are two broad categories of difficult behaviour: non-participation and talking too much. The latter category takes many forms, such as the know-all who always chips in with all the 'answers', people who launch into long stories, people who interrupt, people who do not let other people get a word in edgeways, people who talk off the point, people who always disagree and people who always crack jokes.

A starting point for dealing with these difficulties is to try to think *why* people behave like this. Are they nervous, threatened, worried? Are they desperately in need of attention? If you can deal with the underlying cause, the situation is likely to improve. Secondly, note that people often change their behaviour as they get to know others and feel more comfortable in a group. Thirdly, try getting people to work in pairs or small groups, which can help quiet members to join in, and give others a break from the constant talker. Fourthly, use structures in your discussion such as 'rounds' or make a point of asking for other people's opinions ('Would someone else like to say what he thinks?' 'Would you like to give us your opinion, Ann?'). Finally, it may be necessary to confront the difficult person (not in front of the rest of the group!). For example, you could say: 'I've noticed that you contribute a great deal to the group discussions. That makes me concerned about whether other people are getting enough chance to talk. I'd like to suggest that you keep your comments to just a couple of sentences. Would you feel OK about doing that?'

Notes, References and Further Reading

1 Short courses on working with groups are run by health promotion/education officers in health authorities in various parts of the country.

The Health Education Board for Scotland previously the Scottish Health Education Group has produced a short course on group-work skills:

Wolfe R & Fewell J (1990) *Groupwork Skills: an Introduction*. SHEG: Edinburgh. For further details, including the address of SHEG, see note 3, Chapter Ten

2 See, for example:

Davies M (1984) Training: what we think of it now. *Social Work Today*, **15**(20), 12–17

3 For a general introduction to groupwork, see:

Douglas T (1978) *Basic Groupwork*. London: Routledge & Kegan Paul
Douglas T (1983) *Groups—Understanding People Gathered Together*. London: Routledge & Kegan Paul

Suitable for anyone leading an informal supportive group, of whatever membership:

Houston G (1984) *The Red Book of Groups and How to Lead Them Better*. Available from The Rochester Foundation, 8 Rochester Terrace, London NW1

Suitable particularly for those with a social work background:

Preston-Shoot M (1987) *Effective Groupwork*. British Association of Social Workers Practical Social Work Series. London: Macmillan Education

Suitable for those with a nursing background:

Wright H (1989) *Groupwork: Perspectives and Practice.* London: Scutari Press

Suitable for anyone involved in a self-help project or community group:

Cranwell B (1986) *Get it Together.* Cambridge: National Extension College

Suitable for leaders of support groups:

Nichols C & Jenkinson J (1991) *Leading a Support Group.* London: Chapman & Hall

Suitable for self-help groups:

Gingerbread/CEDC (1990) *Better All Together.* Available from Community Education Development Centre, Lyng Hall, Blackberry Lane, Coventry CV2 3JS. Telephone: 0203 638660

Suitable for anyone facilitating a youth or community group:

Scottish Community Education Council (1987) *100 Good Ideas for Youth and Community Groups.* Available from: Community Education Development Centre, see address above

Suitable for anyone starting and running a community group:

Pinder C (1985) *Community Start Up.* Cambridge: National Extension College.

Suitable for anyone starting or running a voluntary group:

Capper S *et al* (1989) *Starting and Running a Voluntary Group.* London: Bedford Square Press

Suitable for leaders of adult education groups:

Open University (1986) *Leading a Group.* Milton Keynes: Open University

Lever M *et al* (1985) *Learning Together: a Guide to Running Informal Learning Groups.* Cambridge: National Extension College

Henderson P (1989) *Promoting Active Learning.* Cambridge: National Extension College

Suitable for tutors involved in women's education:

Workers' Educational Association (1986) *Working Towards Change.* A training package, available from the Community Education Development Centre (see address above)

Suitable for teachers leading student-centred groups:

Brandes D & Ginnis P (1986) *A Guide to Student-Centred Learning.* Oxford: Basil Blackwell

Baldwin J & Williams H (1988) *Active Learning: a Trainer's Guide.* Oxford: Basil Blackwell

4 Handy C B (1985) *Understanding Organisations.* Harmondsworth: Penguin Business Library, Ch 6

5 Tuckman B W (1965) Developmental sequence in small groups. *Psychological Bulletin*, **63**, 384–399

6 Belbin R M (1981) *Management Teams.* London: Heinemann

7 We acknowledge, with thanks, that much of the material in this section is derived from a checklist produced by Louise Walker and Margaret Douglas, Health Promotion Officers, Bristol & Weston Health Authority, August 1990

8 There are many more 'games' for group leaders in:

Brandes D & Phillips H (1978) *Gamesters Handbook*. London: Hutchinson
Brandes D (1983) *Gamesters Two*. London: Hutchinson

9 Adapted, with kind permission, from:

The Open University, Community Education (1983) *Group Notes*. Open University, p 10

Chapter 10
Helping People to Make Health Choices

Summary

This chapter is about helping people to make health choices. The first section looks at working towards client self-empowerment before outlining strategies for increasing self-awareness, clarifying values and changing attitudes. Strategies for decision-making follow. The chapter ends with principles for using strategies effectively. Exercises, case studies and quizzes are included.

In this chapter we look at the competences you need when you are helping people to make choices about health and to carry them out. Much health behaviour appears to have developed without conscious decision-making; it has 'just happened' in response to individual and group circumstances and external events. *Active* decision-making is different because it involves committing time and effort (yours and your client's) to understanding the factors which influence health choices and behaviour, and to taking considered decisions and actions.[1]

However, it has to be accepted that people may prefer to carry on with behaviour which seems 'unhealthy' to you. To a client, it may not seem 'unhealthy' as the benefits outweigh the risks. Respect for people's right to their own points of view and their own right to choose are fundamental to establishing relationships between health promoters and their clients. (See the first section of Chapter Eight *Exploring relationships with clients* for further discussion of this topic.)

On the other hand, you also have to consider that people's right to individual freedom of choice has to be balanced against the effect of that choice on others; for example, choosing to drink and drive could affect many other people as well as the driver.

Furthermore, choosing a 'healthy' behaviour does not automatically lead to practising it. Changes such as taking more exercise, practising relaxation, going for screening tests, wearing ear protectors in noisy surroundings, eating different foods and stopping smoking are all hard work, and these changes in themselves may be stressful. Social or economic circumstances may also prevent people from carrying out new health behaviours, even if they would like to.

However, despite these limitations, it can be very rewarding to help people to look at their beliefs, values and attitudes, and to make and carry out decisions which will lead to improved health and well-being. We now turn to the strategies and skills you require. (These strategies relate to two of the health promotion aims we discussed in Chapter Six: 'self-empowering' and 'changing attitudes and behaviour'.)

Working for Client Self-empowerment

Making health choices and carrying them out can bring benefits. These are not only the benefits that go with a health-promoting lifestyle, but also increased self-esteem from the feeling of taking active control over a part of life, such as being in control of the smoking habit rather than cigarettes being in control:[2] in other words, making a positive choice about health can be a self-empowering process.

There are a number of different ways of working towards self-empowerment:[3] these include groupwork and experiential learning, individual counselling and therapy, and advocacy. We consider them all in the following sections, except therapy which is beyond the scope of this book. (In any case, unless you are a mental health specialist, most people you work with probably do not need in-depth therapy but could benefit from counselling.)

The process of self-empowering people involves modifying the way people *feel* about themselves through improving their self-awareness and self-esteem. It involves helping them to think critically about their values and beliefs and build up their own values and beliefs system. This is in contrast to traditional teaching which operates largely in the hope that the 'right' attitudes and values will be 'caught' by learners. In the next section, we outline some strategies you may find useful for helping clients to become more self-aware (having greater insight into, and understanding of, themselves, their attitudes and feelings), and to help them clarify their values and attitudes.

Strategies for Increasing Self-awareness, Clarifying Values and Changing Attitudes

Many of the strategies which are useful for increasing self-awareness, clarifying values, developing beliefs systems and changing attitudes are designed for group work (see Chapter Nine). However, some of them can be adapted for health promoters to use in one-to-one situations, to give clients to use by themselves.

They all use the principle of *experiential learning* which emphasises the importance of personal experience as a source of learning.[4] It encourages 'active' learning through undertaking exercises and other activities designed, for example, to increase self-awareness or aid decision-making. Some experiential learning methods are now described.

Ranking or Categorising

Ranking is a way of analysing an issue in order to distinguish the relative importance of different aspects. It is therefore useful for *clarifying values.* For example, in the exercise *What does being healthy mean to you*? in Chapter One readers are asked to rank aspects of 'being healthy'. Health is a value and this exercise is designed to help readers to clarify which aspects of health they value most.

Another approach to *increasing self-awareness and values clarification* is to generate a list of items, and then code them into different categories. The following exercise illustrates this approach; it is designed to raise awareness of the link between enjoyment and health.

Exercise—Enjoyment and health

Quickly list as many things as you can think of that you enjoy doing. Write them down the left-hand side of a piece of paper. On the right-hand side, code each item according to the following categories.

£—any items that involve spending money
A—any items that you do alone
P—any items that you do with other people
R—any items that involve some kind of risk
F—any items that help to keep you fit
C—any items that involve creativity
D—any items that involve consumption of drugs (including alcohol and tobacco)
H+—any items which positively affect your health
H−—any items which negatively affect your health

Items may be coded in more than one category. For example, if one of the things you enjoy is going out to the pub for a drink, this may be coded £, P and D, as well as H+ and/or H−.

What have you learned about enjoyment and health through doing this exercise?

Using Polarised Views

This is a way of getting people to clarify their views about a particular issue. Views about the issue are polarised—that is, phrased to reflect extremely different views. For example, if the issue was 'Is jogging good for you?', polarised views could be summed up as 'Jogging kills people and only very fit athletes should do it' or 'Jogging is very beneficial to health and all people would be fitter if they took it up'. Examples of polarised views can be described by the group leader or taken from writings which express opposite views.

The group leader may ask people to work in pairs, with each individual acting as if he fully adopted one of the points of view for the duration of the exercise, whatever his personal opinions may be. First, each person writes down all the arguments he can think of which support his position, without discussing it with his partner at this stage. After a few minutes, the partners are asked to start arguing their case, usually for about 15 minutes. The leader then lists the points in favour of each view by asking each pair in turn to contribute one point, until all the points have been collected. She then asks the group to comment on what they have learnt. In this way, members of the group can consider a whole range of arguments, which helps them to understand other people's points of view, tolerate differences of opinion, clarify their own views, and perhaps see the issue in a new light.

Another example of a values clarification exercise using the polarised arguments approach is the exercise *Analysing your philosophy of health* promotion in Chapter Three, where readers are asked to consider arguments for and against two polarised views about the aim of health promotion.

Using a Values Continuum

This is an extension of the polarised argument technique. It helps people to understand the spread of opinion on a particular issue, and to clarify where they stand.

The leader describes two extremes of opinion and asks the group to imagine that these can be represented by two points, A and B, joined by a straight line. With a small group this line can be across a room; with a large group it could be drawn on the blackboard. The group members are then asked to mark or place themselves at a point along the line that best reflects their own view. For instance, in the jogging example discussed above, pro-joggers place themselves at one end, with the most extreme at the farthest point, people with moderate views stand around the middle, and the most ardent anti-jogger stands at the other end. The leader asks each person to state his views briefly as he takes up his position. Other people are asked not to interrupt or comment until everyone has taken up a position, or passed if they chose not to participate.

This technique can encourage a more detailed discussion of the range of possible options than the polarised argument technique. On the other hand, if everyone seems moderate, a better discussion may be stimulated by the polarised argument technique.

The values continuum technique is used in the last task of the exercise *Analysing your philosophy of health promotion* in Chapter Three.

Using Role Play

Role play generally means taking on the role of another person in a specified situation, and acting out what that other person might do and say in that situation. This helps people to understand what it feels like to be in another person's shoes. For example, adults role playing an unemployed young person may be helped to understand feelings of rejection and boredom. Health promoters role playing non-English-speaking patients visiting a clinic may be helped to understand how those patients feel, especially if the role play is given added authenticity by using a foreign language which the health promoters do not speak.

It is also possible to role play oneself in a new situation. This is a useful way of practising a new skill or rehearsing for a future event. For example, patients can role play a consultation with a doctor in order to practise the skills of presenting their health problems to doctors.

For an example of role-play exercise,[5] see *Skills of patient education* in Chapter 11.

Playing Games

By *games* we mean structured activities, usually for a group of people, but sometimes for one or two people only. Games are useful for meeting a variety of aims. One is to help people to get to know each other (ice-breakers), such as the name games described in the section *Getting Groups Going* in Chapter Nine. Other games are devised to help people to trust each other, to communicate more openly or to increase self-awareness.[6]

For example, games can be used to help people to identify 'irrational beliefs'. Irrational beliefs are misconceptions which hinder people from achieving their goals.[7] They are usually expressed in terms of 'must', 'should' or 'ought'. There are three major irrational beliefs:[8]

- 'I *must* win everybody's approval otherwise I am worthless'.
- 'Other people *must* treat me exactly how I want them to (and if they don't they must be blamed and punished)'.
- 'Life *must* give me everything I want and nothing I don't want'.

These beliefs lead to self-defeating thinking and this in turn can affect health. It can lead to health-related behaviour with destructive consequences, such as emotional disorders, heavy drinking and physical ailments. The quiz, below, is an example of a game; this one aims to help you to identify your own irrational beliefs.

Exercise—Beliefs quiz

Look at the following statements and put a tick in the appropriate column:

	Agree	Disagree
1. I believe in the saying that "A leopard cannot change his spots".	______	______
2. The more problems people have the less happy they will be.	______	______
3. There are certain 'crisis' points in life when the strain can be too great.	______	______
4. There is more stress and pressure nowadays than when I was a child.	______	______
5. If you try to run a mile when you're over 65 it's bad for your health.	______	______
6. I avoid things I cannot do well.	______	______
7. I feel little anxiety about unexpected dangers or future events.	______	______
8. I believe that 'wait and see' is a good philosophy for life.	______	______
9. I want everyone to like me.	______	______
10. I usually put off important decisions.	______	______

continued on next page

continued

Now identify your rational beliefs and your irrational beliefs (misconceptions):

Q1. If you agreed with this statement you may believe that the past has a lot to do with determining the present and that people are largely unchangeable. 'I'm made that way'. The idea that you are no good at playing sports, for example, can be used to avoid trying out new behaviour and learning the skills necessary to participate in a sport. The truth is that people who take risks, experiment and work on things, generally find that they can become reasonably competent at most of the things they attempt (not necessarily perfect, but good enough).

Q2. If you agreed with this statement you may believe that it is external events that cause human misery and people are victims of whatever fate brings. This is a misconception. In practice there is often much we can do to create our own destiny. Blaming other people or circumstances can be a way of avoiding taking responsibility for ourselves.

Q3. If you agreed with this statement you are right! People who normally cope quite well can get depressed, anxious or ill when faced with major life events such as divorce, redundancy, or the death of a close relative. It isn't a sign of weakness but it is an indication that the person needs support to adjust to the changes.

Q4. This is impossible to answer! It's difficult to measure stress and even more impossible to compare people in different historical periods and circumstances.

Q5. If you agreed with this statement you may hold the belief that exercise is only for the fit, young and healthy. Providing you exercise regularly and sensibly, running a mile when you are over 65 could not only be healthy but enjoyable and good for your self-esteem!

Q6. If you agreed with this statement you may be a bit of a perfectionist. The belief that we are only worth while when we are successful or at least working hard can result in our becoming 'workaholics'. Or it could affect you in the opposite way: not trying out new things for fear of making mistakes or failing. In reality we are all worth while just for being ourselves. If we can break free of this belief we can get more satisfaction from our activities—even when we are not very good at them. And enjoy the easy things as well as struggling with the difficult.

Q7. If you agreed with this statement you have a healthy attitude. Many people experience anxiety and worry over events which are extremely unlikely. They tend to see things as a series of potential catastrophies. 'Wouldn't it be terrible if . . .'. Encourage these people to appreciate how well they handle everyday reality and to develop confidence in their strengths.

Q8. If you agreed with this statement you may believe that human happiness can be achieved by hoping for the best—and waiting to see what happens. This belief could result in you becoming merely a spectator in life—watching television every night and somnolent on a sun-lounger for the whole of your holidays. Getting more actively involved could be more satisfying and actually provide you with more energy. If you feel too 'burnt-out', now may be the time to take a close look at how you are managing your life and make some changes.

continued on next page

continued

Q9. If you agree with this statement you may only believe you are as good as other people think you are. Because of this you may feel worthless if, despite your efforts, people don't seem to like you. Having the approval of others is pleasant, but in order to run our own lives we shall almost certainly have to do some things which some people do not like. Work on giving yourself the approval you deserve.

Q10. If you agreed with this statement you may believe that life's problems will go away if you avoid them. Don't waste your time hoping that things will work out—make them.

Strategies for Decision-Making

As a health promoter, it is likely that you will often be involved in counselling with the aim of helping people to make a choice, such as which treatment to have, whether an elderly person should stay put or move into residential accommodation, whether to have a blood test for HIV or how to select healthy foods in particular circumstances.[9]

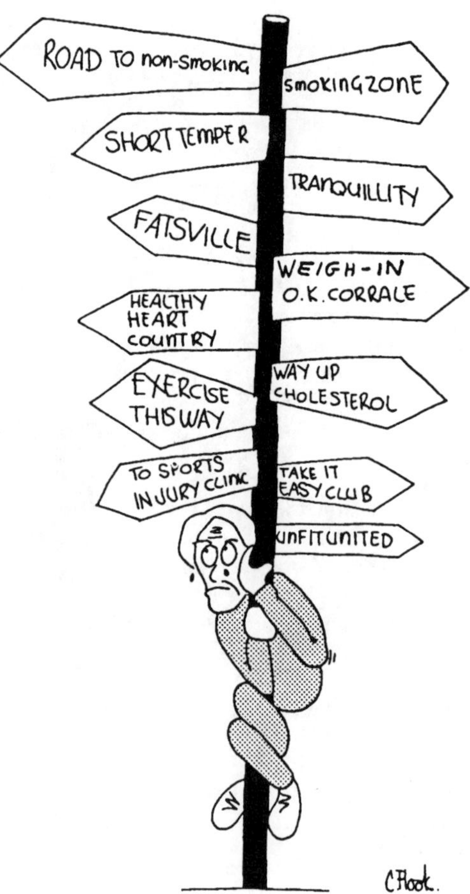

Helping people to make health choices

The *basic skills* of counselling to help people to make decisions are the same as those discussed in Chapter Eight: *understanding non-verbal communication, listening, helping people to talk*, and *asking questions and obtaining feedback*.

There are at least five stages involved.[10] (These stages may seem familiar to you because counselling involves a framework of planning and evaluating similar to the one we used in Chapter Six.)

Stage 1. Identify the need and create the climate

Carl Rogers (a 'founding father' of counselling) has identified the qualities necessary for a counsellor to establish a climate in which a client can 'open up':[11] these are warmth, openness, genuineness, empathy and unconditional positive regard. Unconditional positive regard is the quality of totally respecting the worth and dignity of a person, irrespective of whether you like the person or agree with his views or behaviour.

The practical aspects of creating the climate include ensuring that you will not be interrupted and cannot be overheard, that you have sufficient time, and that you are comfortably seated in chairs of the same height, with the counsellor adopting an open posture and making direct eye contact when appropriate.

Stage 2. Explore the needs and the concerns

Through giving full attention and actively listening, by encouraging the client to talk and by asking questions, the counsellor begins to establish trust and to enable the client to move from superficial issues to deeper needs and concerns.

Stage 3. Help the client to set goals and identify options

Having gained a new perspective on the issues and concerns, it becomes possible for the client to identify goals and ways these might be achieved. The counsellor may help the client to identify themes or to get a clearer vision of the future through asking key questions such as:

'How would you feel if . . . ?'
'If things were exactly how you wanted them to be, how would it be different from now . . . ?'
'Have you ever felt like that on other occasions . . . ?'

The counsellor may also provide the client with information in order to establish options:

'If you do X what's likely to happen is . . .'
'If you do Y the chances are that . . .'
'You might find it helpful to consider that . . .' and so on.

Stage 4. Help the client to decide which option to choose

The important thing about this stage is that the choice must be the client's, not the counsellor's. Making decisions—that is, choosing between alternative options—is a highly complex process. It involves:

- weighing up the pros and cons of the alternative options;

- considering the likely consequences of pursuing each alternative;
- deciding which is the best alternative.

If the client is reluctant to commit himself to a decision, then both parties need to consider whether it is worth undertaking further work at stages two and three. If the client chooses an alternative which the counsellor feels won't work, she should nevertheless back the client's choice and help the client to develop an action plan (knowing that if it doesn't work, the door is still open for exploring other options).

Stage 5. Help the client to develop an action plan

Having made a decision, the client now needs to think about turning that decision into action. He may need to identify coping strategies and sources of support. (See the next section on *Strategies for changing behaviour*.) Once an action plan has been agreed, the final details are to set a review date and to clarify how progress will be monitored.

Example—Counselling about a health choice

A health visitor has the task of helping a mother to decide what to do about having her baby vaccinated. The stages could be:

Stages 1 and 2—Identify and explore the need

For example, is the mother worried about having the child vaccinated at all, or is it just the whooping cough vaccination which is worrying? Is it *when* to have the child vaccinated, or *if*?

Stage 3—Help the client to set goals and establish options

For example, the parent may identify the goal of her child having the best possible chance of staying healthy. The options might be: no vaccinations at all, some vaccinations, or all the vaccinations?

Stage 4—Help the client to decide which option to choose

- Weigh up the pros and cons—the health visitor provides unbiased information on the risk of catching each disease compared with the risk of having the vaccinations.
- Consider the likely consequences of pursuing each alternative: for the child, in terms of health risk; for the parent, in terms of anxiety, guilt and responsibility; for other people, in terms of spreading the diseases.

Stage 5—Help the client to develop an action plan

For example, the mother may decide to go ahead with the vaccination programme, but also to join a mothers' group, in order to get support from other mothers facing the same anxieties and decisions. The health visitor suggests to the mother that she keeps a record of the vaccinations for future reference, and provides her with a record card for her child. They set a date for the first vaccination.

Strategies for Changing Behaviour

Having made a choice, people may need considerable help to carry their decision through into action. A number of techniques developed from behavioural psychology are useful, and the philosophy behind them (that people are responsible for their own behaviour and are capable of exercising control over it) is as important as the techniques themselves.[12] A variety of material has been developed to help people to change different aspects of their behaviour, such as stopping smoking, controlling drinking, changing eating habits and taking up exercise.[13] Some useful techniques are as follows.

Self-monitoring

Self-monitoring is keeping a detailed and precise account, often in the form of a diary, of behaviour which is to be changed. Its aim is to help people to analyse their pattern of behaviour and become fully aware of what they are doing, which is a starting point for gaining control. Secondly, the 'diary' provides a base-line against which progress can be checked.

Self-monitoring involves answering questions such as:

- how frequently does the problem occur?
- when the problem occurs, what else is happening both externally (in the environment), and internally (in thoughts and feelings)?
- what event leads up to the problem?
- what happens afterwards: the consequences?

An example of a Smoker's Diary is given below.

Example of self-monitoring—a smoker's diary

Day . . . . (Complete one of these charts every day)

Each time you smoke a cigarette, note down in the columns:

1 the time
2 how urgent your craving for a cigarette is, on a scale of 1–10 (1 = very little craving, 10 = extremely high craving)
3 where you smoke the cigarette
4 whether you are alone or who you are with
5 do you smoke it with drinks (coffee, tea, alcohol)?
6 do you smoke it after a meal?
7 what else are you doing at the time (eg. chatting, reading the paper, working, talking on the phone)?
8 why did you decide to smoke this cigarette?
9 what do you feel about it afterwards?

Time	Craving	Where	Who with	With drinks	After meal	Doing what	Why	Afterwards

Total number of cigarettes smoked today = ______

Identifying Costs, Benefits and Rewards

The cost of changing behaviour can be considerable, involving deprivation of 'crutches', such as cigarettes, and pleasures, such as eating and drinking, or there may be a heavy price to pay in terms of time, effort and perhaps money. So it is helpful to identify the benefits clearly, and set up a system of rewards to encourage perseverance.

Benefits may be long-term, such as better health or increased life-expectancy. They may be abstract ('It will prove I've got will-power') or in other people's interests ('for the family's sake'). Important though these benefits may be, it is also necessary to find immediate, short-term rewards which people genuinely enjoy, such as small treats.[14]

Setting Targets and Evaluating Progress

Targets should be realistic rather than idealistic. Losing an average of one pound in weight a week is realistic for most people; losing a stone in a month usually is not. People may have unrealistic hopes and expectations about what can be achieved, which leads to disappointment and a sense of failure when the target has not been met.

In order to evaluate progress, it is necessary to keep a record of behaviour so that achievements can be seen clearly. Progress should be assessed once the 'new' behaviour has been given a fair trial perhaps for two or three weeks, although short-term reviews ('How have I done today?') can also be useful.

If the target is not being achieved, possible reasons must be looking for and changes made. For example:

- is the target too difficult? Should it be lowered?
- are the rewards too distant? Is there a more immediate reward which could be more encouraging?
- is there an unforeseen crisis or illness? If so, encouragement to continue self-monitoring and to look on the setback as a learning experience may be needed.
- are other people unhelpful? More strategies to cope with the negative influence of other people may be needed.
- are there other problems which require help, such as learning to cope with anxiety or stress?

Devising Coping Strategies

Changing behaviour can mean coping with numerous difficulties, for at least a short period of time, until the new behaviour becomes a normal part of life. Someone who is stopping smoking has to cope with problems such as the craving he feels, the need to put something in his mouth, not knowing what to do with his hands, doing without his accustomed 'tension-reliever' in moments of stress, and resisting the offer of a cigarette.

People adopt a wide variety of coping strategies, and it is often useful to get a group to share their ideas about what helps them to cope.[15] The list of strategies here is certainly not exhaustive:

- finding a substitute, such as substituting chewing gum or herbal cigarettes for the real thing, or eating low-calorie foods instead of high-calorie ones;
- changing some routines and habits which are closely associated with the 'problem'

behaviour. Examples are drinking tea or fruit juice instead of coffee, because coffee is closely associated with cigarettes;

- making it difficult to carry on with the 'problem' behaviour, by, for example, keeping cigarettes in an inconvenient place, sitting in a no-smoking compartment, and deciding to restrict eating to mealtimes, not between meals.

What all these strategies have in common is that they require only a small step to achieve a large degree of help for self-control. Other strategies may be:

- getting support from other people in the same boat, who might be from a slimming group, an anti-smoking clinic, or a self-help group. Another helpful way of getting support is by linking with another person on the understanding that each may telephone or meet the other if either of them needs help[16] (see Chapter Nine for further reading on self-help groups).
- practising ways of responding to unhelpful social pressures, for example, refusing the offer of a cigarette or a drink.
- adopting a one-day-at-a-time approach. The prospect of the whole of the rest of life without a cigarette may be overwhelming, but the prospect of one day without one is far more tolerable. Even shorter time-spans may be helpful, such as putting off eating, drinking or smoking for just five minutes at a time.
- learning relaxation techniques and other ways (such as exercise) of relieving stress. Simple relaxation routines which can be practised at any time and place can be helpful in coping with stressful moments when the 'old' reaction would have been to reach for a drink or a cigarette.

Case study—Changing behaviour in practice

Joan is divorced. She has a toddler who constantly wakes her at night. She has used various stratagems, including trying to tire him out physically just before bedtime, keeping him up later, leaving toys for him to play with in the night, and playing with him herself in the night. She has started to have a few glasses of sherry in the evenings to help her to relax and now finds that she needs another sherry to help her get back to sleep after getting up in the night.

She goes to her doctor for help. He explains that the strategems she used to try to get her son to sleep do not work because they merely stimulate him and give him rewards (playing and getting attention from his mother) when he wakes up. He suggests that the toddler needs to learn to relax before he goes to bed. The doctor asks Joan if she knows anything which seems to help her child to relax, and using her suggestions they devise a suitable bedtime routine for Joan to try out.

Turning to Joan herself, the doctor asks how she has been coping and Joan responds that a few sherries in the evening helped at first but now she is worried that she may be relying too much on drinking to help her to cope. He then asks about her reasons for drinking. She has already identified that it helps her to cope; it makes her feel less anxious and 'strung up'. She says 'When I've had a hard day I deserve a drink . . . it helps me relax and forget my problems for a while'.

continued on next page

continued

The doctor asks her to think of reasons why drink may not be the most helpful way to reward herself, help herself to relax or solve her problems. He suggests that she should think about alternatives, such as leisure activities. He tells her about a local mother-and-toddler group where she can meet other mothers in similar circumstances. He suggests that she keeps a drinker's diary so that they can together find out more about her drinking patterns and help her to set limits on her drinking. He shows her an example of a drinker's diary and explains how to count each drink using standard measures. Joan agrees to fill it in every time she has a drink during the next fortnight.

Finally, he asks Joan to come back and see him in two weeks' time to discuss whether the new routines are helping the toddler to sleep and to see what she has discovered from the suggestions he has made. He also arranges for the health visitor to visit Joan in a few days' time.

What strategies does the doctor use to help Joan with her problems? What other strategies could he have used?

Using Strategies Effectively

We have discussed a number of different strategies which you can use when you are trying to help clients to increase their self-awareness, clarify their values and beliefs, and change their attitudes and behaviour. In order to use these strategies with maximum effect there are a number of principles to bear in mind.

Advocacy

Some people may need extra help to make health choices. *Advocacy* is generally taken to mean representing the interests of people who cannot speak up for themselves because of illness, handicap or other disadvantage. In the context of health promotion, it is better seen as a variety of ways of empowering those people who are disempowered in our society. It is concerned with using every possible means to assist people to become independent and *self-advocating*.

There can be deep conflicts of loyalty for health promoters who take on an advocacy role, for it may be necessary to challenge employers, or those in authority, about services which fail to meet people's needs. For example, if a patient complains to a community psychiatric nurse that his drugs are making him feel drowsy and generally unwell, but the doctor insists he should continue to take them, where should the nurse's loyalties lie: to the patient, to the doctor, to the Health Authority (which employs her) or to the profession (which controls her registration)? How can the nurse most effectively act as an advocate in this situation?

Because of these conflicts of loyalty, many advocacy schemes use non-professional workers who come from a similar background to those they are empowering. For example, 'Maternity Links' schemes provide workers as advocates and interpreters for Asian mothers who do not speak English. The workers are Asian themselves, able to speak English as well as their mother tongue, and the organisation may be run with health authority funding but managed independently.

Making Healthier Choices Easy Choices

People do not make health choices in a vacuum; they make them in the context of their own environment, subject to all the pressures and influences that surround them. If this environment is conducive to a healthier lifestyle, clients have greater freedom to choose the 'healthier' alternatives and change their behaviour. For example, the provision of cycleways makes it easier to take regular exercise by cycling to work; provision of litter bins, combined with frequent emptying, helps people to Keep Britain Tidy; a no-smoking policy in public places such as restaurants and cinemas helps people not to smoke. National and local policies can create a climate where it is easier to adopt healthier behaviour. (See the section *What affects health?* in Chapter One and Chapter 13 *Changing Policy and Practice.*)

Relating to Clients

Research consistently shows that the degree of client change is related to helper empathy; in other words, clients are more likely to change if the health promoter understands the client, sees things from his point of view, and accepts him on his own terms (this has been discussed at more length in the section in Chapter Eight *Relationships with clients*). Achieving this relationship may be the most difficult part of helping people to change. Furthermore, the attitude and behaviour of the health promoter herself is likely to influence the outcome. For example, doctors who themselves smoke are less likely to be effective in helping people to choose to stop smoking.[17]

Using Learning Methods Sensitively

People invest a great deal of emotion in their values and attitudes, which means that the exercises we have described here, especially those that are designed to encourage people to explore feelings, such as role-play, need to be handled with care and sensitivity. Special training in the use of experiential teaching methods is recommended, but at the very least, group leaders should not attempt to use them unless they have experienced them first themselves. Some points to remember are as follows.

- Explain the activities carefully and thoroughly, and check to ensure that everybody understands what the exercise is for, and what they are expected to do.
- Emphasise that participation is entirely voluntary.
- Allow plenty of time for discussion at the end. If people's opinions and cherished ideas have been challenged, they are likely to feel strongly about it. Increased self-awareness may be a very uncomfortable experience, too. The group leader should ensure that people have time to express their feelings and get any support that they need before they leave the group.
- Ensure that there is an atmosphere of confidentiality and trust, so that people feel free to explore their views and feelings in safety. If they feel they may be laughed at or gossiped about, they will not participate fully, if at all.
- Save your own views to the end, after the group members have had a chance to think things through for themselves. Be open and honest about yourself and your values, and if you, too, are confused, say so!

Taking a Long-term View

Changes in attitude and behaviour may take a long time, and single sessions by health promoters are unlikely to have much effect, unless they are part of a long-term strategy. Follow-up work is very important. For example, evaluation of the Give Up Smoking (GUS) kits designed to assist general practitioners to help patients to stop smoking, suggests that those GPs who make follow-up appointments are more likely to be effective.[18]

Notes, References and Further Reading

1 For reading on the theory of attitude change, decision-making and behaviour change, and the links between them, see:

Eiser J R & Vander Pligt J (1988) *Attitudes and Decisions.* London: Routledge & Kegan Paul (see particularly the section on health)

Tones K, Tilford S & Robinson Y (1990) *Health Education—Effective and Efficiency.* London: Chapman & Hall, Ch 3

2 For an example see the study:

Langer E J & Rodin J (1976) The effects of choice and enhanced social responsibility: a field experiment in an institutional setting. *Journal of Personal & Social Pscyhology*, **34**, 191–198. This study showed that residents in a home for the elderly who were given personal responsibility and choice showed improved alertness, active participation and self-rated well-being when compared with control subjects.

3 For a consideration of the wide range of intervention skills required, see:

Burnard P (1985) *Learning Human Skills: a Guide for Nurses.* Oxford: Heinemann Nursing

4 Experiential learning has evolved from two sources. One is from the theories of the American philosopher John Dewey. Another is from humanistic psychology. Humanistic psychology sees people as free decision-makers, actively controlling their own destinies. We have already discussed some limitations to this viewpoint in Chapter Three, but humanistic psychology has had a huge influence on health care, education and health promotion both in this country and worldwide. The literature is vast, but for interested readers we suggest starting by reading Philip Burnard's *Learning Human Skills*, Ch 2 (see reference 3, above).

5 See:

Evans M, Rice W & Grey G (1981) *Free to Choose—an Approach to Drug Education.* Salford: TACADE, Section 7—A Visit to the Doctor

6 For many 'games' for group leaders to use, see:

Brandes D & Phillips H (1978) *Gamesters Handbook.* London: Hutchinson

Brandes D (1983) *Gamesters Two.* London: Hutchinson

7 For a discussion on the role of irrational beliefs, see:

Trower P, Casey A & Dryden W (1988) *Cognitive-Behavioural Counselling in Action*. London: Sage Publications, Ch 1

8 Ellis A (1980) An Overview of the Clinical Theory of Rational-Emotive Therapy. In Grieger R & Boyd J (eds) *Rational-Emotive Therapy: a Skills-based Approach*. New York: Van Nostrand Reinhold

For an approach to counselling based on rational-emotive therapy, see:

Dryden W (1987) *Counselling Individuals: The Rational-Emotive Approach*. London: Taylor & Francis

9 For further reading on counselling, see:

Dass R & Gorman P (1985) *How can I help?* London: Rider Books
Nelson-Jones R (1988) *Practical Counselling and Helping Skills: Helping Clients to Help Themselves*. London: Cassell Educational

The Health Education Board for Scotland, previously the Scottish Health Education Group (SHEG) have produced a guide for those wishing to set up and run short introductory counselling courses for nurses, midwives and health visitors:

SHEG (1990) *Sharing Counselling Skills: a Guide to Running Courses for Nurses, Midwives and Health Visitors*. Available from The Health Education Board for Scotland, Woodburn House, Canaan Lane, Edinburgh EH10 4SG

The Health Education Board for Scotland (formerly SHEG) in Edinburgh have also produced a series of six modular courses in counselling and helping skills, which are designed to be used separately or in combination:

Carruthers T (1991) *Initial Interviewing and Assessment Skills*
Woolfe R (1991) *Counselling Skills: a Training Manual*
Robinson F & Robson K (1991) *Problem Identification and Personal Problem Solving*
Woolfe R & Fewell J (1991) *Groupwork Skills: an Introduction*
Evison R (1991) *Personal and Intra-agency Support and Supervision*
Cherry C, Roberson M & Meadows F (1991) *Personal and Professional Development for Group Leaders*

The Health Education Board for Scotland also runs a telephone information service on where to find counselling services and counselling training in Scotland. Telephone: 031 452 8989

For counselling training for those working with HIV/AIDS, contact:

Counselling Support and Health, 105 Hinton Way, Gt Shelford, Cambridge CB2 5AJ

See also:

SHEG (1989) *HIV/AIDS: Counselling Skills for the General Practitioner*. A videotape plus training notes, available from The Health Education Board for Scotland, address as above.

10 Philip Burnard (see Reference 2 above) identifies 8 stages. We have adapted our 5 stages from Burnard, and from:

Inskipp F (1986) *Counselling: The Trainer's Handbook.* Cambridge: National Extension College

11 Rogers C R (1983) *Freedom to Learn For the Eighties.* Columbus, Ohio: Charles E Mervil

12 For a general introduction to behaviour theory and self-control methods, see:

Watson D L & Tharp R G (1985) *Self-Directed Behaviour—Self-Modification for Personal Adjustment.* Monterey, CA: Brooks/Cole

Kanfer F H & Goldstein A P (1986) *Helping People Change.* Oxford: Pergamon Press

13 For examples, see the Health Promotion/Education Department of your local health authority.

14 Self-rewarding ideas are included in 'Changing Your Ways?' in the *Look After Yourself, Community Education Study Package* Discussion Pack (for individual study). A group pack for use with groups of up to six people is also available. Open University, Walton Hall, Milton Keynes MK7 6AA

15 Many coping strategies are listed in leaflets from the Health Education Authority and the Health Education Board for Scotland, which deal with the relevant aspect of behaviour change such as stopping smoking or drinking more sensibly.

16 For example, pairs who contact each other between group meetings are more likely to be successful at ceasing to smoke than pairs who do not. See:

Janis I L *et al* (1970) Facilitating effects of daily contact between partners who make a decision to cut down on smoking. *Journal of Personal & Social Psychology*, **17**, 25–35

17 Pincherle G *et al* (1970) Smoking habits of business executives: doctor variations in reducing consumption. *Practitioner*, **205**, 209–212

18 Health Education Council *Give Up Smoking* kits for General Practitioners

Chapter 11
Teaching and Instructing

Summary

The first section of this chapter uses an exercise to analyse the qualities and abilities of a good teacher, and then outlines some principles of effective teaching. Subsequent sections contain guidelines on giving talks, strategies for patient education and on teaching practical skills. A role-play exercise on skills of patient education is included.

This chapter is about the skills and methods of traditional teaching, when the aims are primarily educational, concerned with helping people to acquire knowledge or skills. Examples of these are giving a talk on a health topic to a large community group, running an adult education class in food hygiene and safety, giving information to a patient about his diagnosis, treatment and self-care, teaching a small group of colleagues about the techniques and procedures used in a screening programme, or instructing a patient how to test his own urine samples for sugar.

We have focused on selected aspects of education and learning which we identify as specially relevant for health promoters. This chapter is certainly not comprehensive, and further reading is recommended.[1] Other chapters also contain relevant material, especially Chapters Six, Eight, Nine and Ten.

Health promoters generally have credibility because of their training and expert knowledge. This is likely to be valued and respected by clients, but expertise alone does not make a good teacher. The next section is concerned with identifying the qualities and skills of a good teacher.

What Makes a Good Teacher?

Every health promoter has spent many hours on the receiving end of other people's teaching, and this in itself is a useful learning experience. The following exercise will help health promoters to identify factors which have helped and hindered their own learning, and to assess their own qualities and abilities.

Exercise—What helps and hinders learning?

Think of two occasions when you have been a learner, such as when you were a student in class, or in the audience listening to a talk, or when you were being taught on a one-to-one basis. These occasions need not have been connected with work (for example, listening to an art lecture or taking a driving lesson). One should be when you felt, overall, that the teaching session was *good* and the other when it was *bad*. The aim of the exercise is to identify the factors that made them good or bad for you.

In each of your two situations in turn, identify factors which helped you to learn, and factors which hindered your learning. Think of these factors in three categories:

- factors to do with *the environment* (eg. too hot? noisy? hard chairs? a spacious, comfortable room?)
- factors to do with *the qualities of the teacher herself* (eg. sense of humour? appeared bored? contagious enthusiasm? seemed unfriendly?)
- factors to do with *the presentation* (eg. talked too long? used relevant illustrations? involved audience? muddled? used words you didn't understand? used audiovisual aids effectively?)

Enter these factors in on chart:

	Environment	Teacher	Presentation
Factors which helped			
Factors which hindered			

If you are working in a group, compare your chart with those of other people.
What have you learnt about the importance of the environment?
What qualities of a good teacher do you think you already possess?
What helpful points about presentation do you think you already use in your own teaching?
What points about your own qualities or presentation would you like to improve?

We do not suggest that health promoters set out to change their personalities. The aim of identifying strengths and weaknesses is to provide a basis for developing skills.

Some Principles of Effective Teaching

Here we identify some basic principles which should be borne in mind in all teaching, whether to individuals or groups.

Work from the Known to the Unknown

Your starting point is what people know already; this is obvious common sense, but frequently overlooked. The result is that time is wasted by teaching people what they already know, or by talking over their heads. You need to find out as much as possible about what your clients already know. If you cannot do this in advance, spend some time at the beginning of the session asking a few questions. If you have a mixed audience with varying degrees of knowledge, it may be best to acknowledge that some people know more than others, and you will have to make a decision about the level at which to pitch your information: 'Some of you will probably know this, but I'll talk about it briefly because it will be new to others . . .'.

Your aim is build new information, or new skills, on to what is already known.

Aim for Maximum Involvement

People learn best if they are actively involved in the learning process, not just passively listening.

First, try to involve your clients in deciding the aim and content of the teaching. If you are running a course, such as a series of antenatal classes or one on food hygiene, you might begin by explaining your aims, asking for comments and suggestions, and then going on to discuss the content. This will help to increase motivation by including clients' own interests and, hopefully, stimulating them to think about new areas. It also helps clients to recognise that they are responsible for their own learning. The goals and content of one-to-one teaching can always be established by mutual agreement at the beginning of a session.

As a general rule, it is worth considering how much room for negotiation there is in your teaching, and spending time to find out what people really want. Ask yourself: 'Is what I teach what *I want to teach* or what *my clients want to learn*?'

Secondly, keep your clients involved as much as possible during teaching sessions. This is a challenge if you are giving a talk or a lecture to a large audience, but there are possibilities, such as asking people to respond to a question, eg. 'I'd like you to put your hand up if you made a New Year resolution to take more exercise this year'. Or ask them to respond to a series of statements: for example, as an introduction to a talk on nutrition, ask the audience to stand up, then ask them to sit down if they: usually eat white bread . . . add sugar to tea and coffee . . . regularly eat fried food . . . add salt at the table . . . Most of them will be sitting down by now but they will feel alert and involved. Another way of keeping an audience involved is to give them time to talk. This can be done by having question-and-answer sessions, or by allowing short breaks when they can talk about something in groups of two or three for a few minutes. In a talk on passive smoking, for example, you could give your audience a couple of minutes to tell their neighbours how they are affected by other people's smoke.

You can also keep people involved with eye contact. Look members of your audience in the eye, and make sure that you look round at everybody, not just the people immediately in front of you.

Vary your Teaching Methods

It is natural to consider teaching from the teacher's point of view but it may be more helpful to look at it from the client's point of view. For example, talking for half an hour demands concentrated effort and total involvement on your part; but all your audience is doing is listening, which only involves one of their senses and is highly unlikely to hold their full attention for that length of time.

Bringing variety into health teaching can be done in many ways—these include strategies that can be used with individuals, groups, large audiences, children or adults.

Client involvement	*Materials and methods*
Listen	Lectures, audiotapes
Read	Books, booklets, leaflets, handouts, posters, black/white board, flipchart, overhead projector transparency
Look	Photographs, drawings, paintings, posters, charts, material from magazines (such as advertisements), flannelgraphs
Look and listen	Films, videotapes, tape-slide sets, slides with commentary, demonstrations
Listen and talk	Question-and-answer sessions, discussions, informal conversations, debates, brainstorming
Read, listen and talk	Case studies, discussions based on study questions or handouts
Read, listen, talk and actively participate	Drama, role-play, games, simulations, quizzes, practising skills
Read and actively participate	Programmed learning, computer-assisted learning
Make and use	Models, charts, drawings
Use	Equipment
Action research	Gathering information, opinions, interviews and surveys
Projects	Making health education materials—videos, leaflets etc
Visits	To health service premises, fire station, sewage works, play groups, voluntary organisations
Write	Articles, letters to the press, stories, poems

(For discussion of some of these methods, see Chapters Nine and Ten; for discussion on the use of audiovisual aids, see Chapter 14.)

Ensure Relevance

When teaching you should ensure that, as far as possible, what you say is relevant to the needs, interests, and circumstances of the clients. For example, recommendations about health-promoting activities which cost money may be helpful to a relatively well-off audience, but not of much use to an audience which has no money for 'extras'. A discussion on vaccination may be irrelevant to a pregnant woman whose overwhelming concern is the birth itself; she may not relate to an issue which will not affect her until afterwards.

You will help your clients to see the relevance of your subject if you use concrete examples, practical problems and case studies to explain and illustrate your points. Abstract generalisations and quotations of huge figures are difficult to relate to. For example say 'one person in ten' instead of 'X million people in this country', tell the story of a home accident rather than describe a list of risk factors, and describe 'increasing the risk' by saying 'It's like driving a car with faulty brakes—there's no guarantee that you will have an accident, but your chances of having one are greater'.

Identify Realistic Goals and Objectives

We have already discussed (in Chapter Six) the importance of clearly identifying health promotion aims and objectives but it is worth emphasising again how essential it is to be clear about what you are trying to do (raise awareness of a health issue? give people more health knowledge?) and what you want your clients to know, feel and/or do at the end of your teaching session. As we mentioned above, your clients may be involved in these decisions.

A common mistake is to attempt too much. Three or four key points is all that you can ever expect people to remember from a teaching session. Teaching more than that does not mean that they learn more; it usually means that they forget more. For example, if you are asked to give a talk on a huge theme, such as Food for Health, Avoiding Accidents, First Aid or Pollution, you will need to select what you feel to be the few points most relevant for your audience, and avoid the temptation to give an everything-you-ever-wanted-to-know-about talk. A well-moved molehill is better than an abortive attempt to shift Everest.

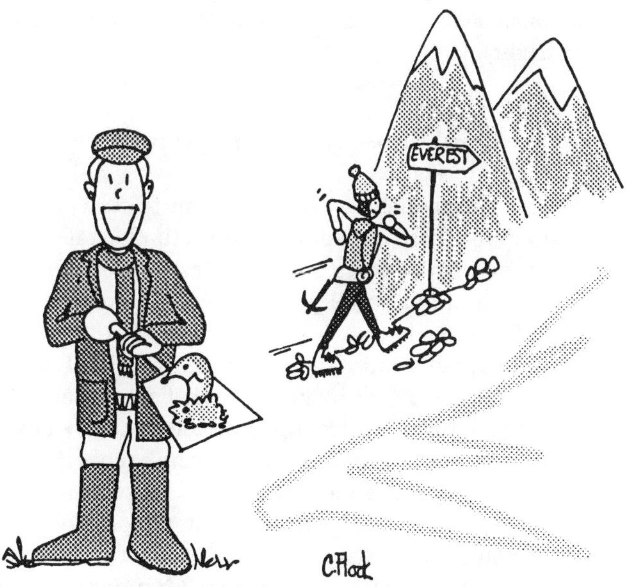

A common mistake is attempting too much . . . a well-moved molehill is better than an abortive attempt to shift Everest

Organise your Material

Whether you are talking to a group or teaching an individual, it helps if you organise your material into a logical framework, and tell your client(s) what this is, both at the beginning, and during, your teaching session.

For example, with an individual patient, say:

'I am going to tell you:
- what we have found to be wrong with you;
- the treatment I am going to suggest for you;
- how much time you will need off work.

First, what we have found out is that . . .
Secondly, I think that the best treatment for you is . . .
Finally, about taking time off work, I think that you will probably need . . .'

The same principle applies if you are talking to a group. The old adage is: 'Tell 'em what you're going to tell 'em; tell 'em; then tell 'em what you've told 'em'. This is sound advice, because it helps both you and the audience to know where you are and where you are going. 'Flagging' where you are at intervals is helpful: 'That's all I've got to say on the benefits of yoga; now, to move on to how you can get started . . .', or 'Now I'd like to move on to my third and final point, which you may remember I said was about . . .'.

Evaluation and Feedback

It is important to get feedback on your teaching, so that you can assess how much your client is learning and improve your own performance in the future (see the section *Stage 5 Plan evaluation methods* in Chapter Six and that on *Asking questions and getting feedback* in Chapter Eight).

Guidelines for Giving Talks

Giving a talk, or perhaps a formal lecture, is a frequent feature of a health promoter's work. There are considerable disadvantages in this method: a talk is largely a one-way communication process with little opportunity to assess how much people are learning or understanding, and with only a small proportion of it likely to be remembered at the end and still less a few days later.

Despite these limitations, talks and lectures can be valuable for several reasons. A talk can be used to introduce a subject by giving a bird's-eye view of it, and this may lead people to take further action. For example, an introductory talk on first aid may lead people to enrol for a first-aid course. A talk may awaken a critical attitude in the audience, for example, by drawing their attention to issues such as pollution or the lack of understandable information on food labels. Many people do not read books and articles or habitually watch documentary programmes on television; for them, a talk may be an important source of health information. Giving talks is also a relatively economical way to use a health promoter's time, since large numbers of people can be addressed at one time.

In addition to the general principles discussed in the last section there now follow some specific points which may help you to plan, and deliver, a successful talk.[3]

Check the Facilities

If possible, visit the place where you are going to give your talk, and check the seating, lighting and audiovisual equipment including electric power points and extension leads. On the day of the talk, arrive in good time so that you can arrange chairs, open windows, put up blackout and check that the equipment is working. Get your video player, overhead projector, slide or film projector ready for use, and if you need blackout, check that you can turn the lights on and off quickly so that you do not lose rapport with the audience while they are left in the dark.

Making and Using Notes

It is generally best to give a talk from notes written on paper or cards. The more experienced you are the fewer notes you are likely to need, unless your talk is full of technical detail or likely to be taken down and quoted verbatim (eg. by the press). However, very few people can give a successful talk with no notes at all, and beginners may find it helpful to write out a talk in full before they transfer the main points to notes.

If you are writing out your talk in full to begin with, it is useful to know that a 50 minute lecture consists of about 5,000 words, allowing for pauses and an estimated speed of delivery of about 110 words per minute. You can then try transferring the key points as notes to cards or paper.

Never give a talk by writing it out in full and then reading it. Unless you are an exceptional orator who can 'act' the lines, it will sound flat and stilted. Furthermore, you will find difficulty in looking at your audience, because you will need to keep your eyes on the notes, and once you look up you are likely to lose your place.

Prepare your Introduction

Secure the attention of your audience with your opening words. Some ways of doing this are:

- state a startling fact;
- ask a question which has no easy answer;
- use a visual image to trigger interest;
- get the audience to do something active (some suggestions are discussed in the earlier section on *Aiming for maximum involvement*);
- tell a joke, if you have the confidence to do it successfully.

Establish eye contact with your audience and, if necessary, ask them if they can see and hear you.

State your aim and theme at the beginning of your talk ('Tell 'em what you're going to tell 'em'). It should be a brief statement, not a complex summary of the whole talk. For example, say 'I'm going to talk about what to do if someone is unconscious, not breathing, bleeding or in a state of shock' but do not go into detail at this point about what the correct actions should be; save that for the main part of the talk.

By the time you have finished the introduction, you should have:

- established your aim and theme with the audience;
- obtained their interest and commitment;
- ensured that they can hear and see you clearly.

Prepare the Key Points

Identify the three or four main points you wish to make, and prepare your talk around each point in turn. Illustrate and support your points with evidence from your experience or from research, with examples, audiovisual materials, and so on. (See Chapter 14 on using and producing audiovisual materials, including leaflets, handouts, films and slides.)

Plan a Conclusion

You need to plan how you will end your talk in order to avoid rambling on or trailing off. Some ways of ending are:

- a very brief recapitulation (not a boring repetition) of what you've said—'We've now covered the basics of life-saving first aid'.
- a statement of what you hope the audience will do with the information you have given them—'I hope that you can confidently do the right thing next time you have to help someone who's had an accident'.
- a suggestion for further action—'If you'd like to learn more please come to see me afterwards'.
- a question—'Don't you think that basic first aid is so simple and so important that it should be taught to every child in school?'
- thank the audience for their attention and/or participation.

Ask for Questions

If possible, include a question-and-answer session in your talk. It gives you feedback, and gives the audience a chance to participate.

When you ask for questions, allow people time to think; do not assume that there are to be no questions just because one is not instantly forthcoming. When a question is asked, it is often helpful to repeat or summarise it. This gives you a little time to consider the question, and ensures that everyone else in the audience has heard it. Never ignore or refuse to answer a question—if you don't know the answer say so, and ask if anyone else in the audience does. In any case, this helps to involve the audience; you could also ask for comments on answers 'Does anyone else have suggestions which could help the lady who asked that question?'

Work on your Presentation

Important points about presentation include pace and timing, which usually means having consciously to slow down your rate of speaking; the nervous beginner finds the silence of pauses to be threatening and wants to get the whole thing over! Other factors are looking at the audience and using notes appropriately.

Thorough preparation will help you to feel confident, but however nervous or inexperienced you may feel, do not apologise for being there. For example, if you have been asked to give a talk about your work, *do not* say 'I'm going to talk about the work of health visitors, but I'm afraid I've only been qualified for a year so there's a lot I don't know yet'. Instead, present yourself positively 'I'm going to talk about the work of health visitors. I've been qualified for a year now, and I'd like to share my experience of the work with you'.

The way to improve presentation is by practice. Practise giving your talk out loud, or to friends or colleagues. Ask a trusted colleague to sit in when you give a talk, and to give you feedback afterwards. It is even more helpful to see yourself on videotape, so that you can assess your own strengths and weaknesses.

Plan for Contingencies

A major fear when giving a talk is that you may 'dry up' or lose your place. If this is a possibility, it is better to face it and think beforehand about what you will do if it should happen. It is best to acknowledge that you have a problem rather than leave an embarrassed silence. For example, say 'Sorry, my mind seems to have gone blank' or 'I've lost my place'. Then remember that an audience is likely to be friendly rather than hostile and will probably want to help you. So let them help by asking for time: 'Would you mind if I took a minute to get myself together' or 'Excuse me for a moment while I look through my notes'.

Another fear is that audiovisual equipment will break down. You cannot insure against this, so it is best to have a contingency plan ready. For example, 'As we can't see the sequence on the film as I'd hoped, I'll write the stages up on the blackboard and talk through them instead' (see also the section *Dealing with difficulties* in Chapter Nine).

Improving Patient Education

Research over many years has shown that patients want information but have difficulty in understanding and remembering what they have been told by their doctor, nurse or other health worker. Substantial numbers of patients feel dissatisfied with the communications aspect of their encounters with health professionals, and are reluctant to ask for more information even when they would very much like it. Furthermore, a large proportion of patients do not comply with the advice and treatment prescribed for them.[4]

There are many reasons for these apparent failures, but certainly some of the cause lies in the way in which information, advice and instructions are given to patients. Often the circumstances are less than ideal, because patients are distressed or feeling unwell, and there may be little time in a busy surgery or outpatient clinic. Therefore, there is all the more reason to ensure that the best possible use is made of the time and opportunities for patient education.

All the basic communication skills discussed in Chapter Eight, and the principles of effective teaching outlined earlier in the present chapter, are important. In addition, there are some particular principles which have been found helpful in patient education.[5]

Some Principles of Patient Education

Say important things first: patients are more likely to remember what was said at the beginning of a session, so give the most important advice and instruction first whenever possible.

Stress and repeat the key points: patients are more likely to remember what they consider to be important, so make sure they realise what the really important points are. For example, say:

'The *most important* thing for you to remember today is . . .'
'The one thing it's really *essential* to do is . . .'

Repetition of key points also helps people to remember them.

Give specific, precise advice: sometimes it is appropriate to give general guidance, but specific, precise advice is more likely to be remembered than vague guidance. For example, say:

'I advise you to lose five pounds in the next month' rather than 'I advise you to lose weight'
'Try to take an hour's rest with your feet up every afternoon' rather than 'Get more rest' or 'Take things easier'.

Structure information into categories: this means telling the patient headings and then categorising your material under these headings as you present it. (See section four *Organise your material* above.)

Avoid jargon and long words and sentences: if you need to use medical terms or jargon, make sure the patient understands what they mean. Never use a long word when a short one will do. Use short sentences.

Use visual aids, leaflets, handouts and written instructions: see Chapter 14 *Using and Producing Health Promotion Materials*.

Avoid saying too much at once: three or four key points is all that you can expect someone to remember from one session.

Ensure that your advice is relevant and realistic in the patient's circumstances: see section *Ensure relevance* above.

Get feedback from patients to ensure that they understand: see section *Asking questions and getting feedback* in Chapter Eight.

The following exercise is designed to help you to practise the skills of patient education discussed here, as well as the basic communication skills outlined in Chapter Eight. Another useful way of learning to improve communication skills is to video and analyse an interview with a patient.[6] Suggestions for further study on patient education are given at the end of this chapter.[7]

Teaching Practical Skills

Health promoters are often called upon to teach practical skills, such as relaxation or keep-fit exercises, how to bath a baby or change a nappy, and how to give an injection or test urine.

All the communication skills we have discussed are relevant, but a few additional points are useful. Teaching a skill is not just about achieving 'knowing' and 'doing' objectives; that is, it is not *solely* concerned with giving the client information and teaching new practical skills. It is also necessary to pay attention to what clients *feel*. If people are afraid to do something because they are worried about looking foolish or doing it incorrectly, they are unlikely to succeed: encouragement and step-by-step progress is needed. Confidence-building is as important a part of the health educator's role as developing practical skills.

In order to develop clients' ability to perform a skilled task, a three-stage approach is most effective, namely:

- demonstrate
- rehearse
- practise

Clients will be watching and listening in stage 1, but they become actively involved in *doing* in stages 2 and 3.

It may be useful to begin by using a dummy, for example, when teaching safe lifting techniques, or to use an orange instead of a person when teaching injection techniques. As skills develop, the techniques can be tried in real life situations (lifting people, for example) and perhaps under more difficult circumstances.

Individual learners need to progress at their own pace and build up confidence at each stage. For this reason teaching practical skills needs time and patience, but it is worth the investment to get the right skills programme from the beginning. People who have lost confidence in their ability to do something are even more difficult to help than a new learner.

Exercise—Skills of patient education

Work in groups of three, taking each role in turn.

The *first person* takes the role of the health promoter. She selects the topic to be taught, drawing on her own experience, and tells the 'patient' his medical history before role-play starts.

The *second person* plays the patient. This patient has one of the following sets of characteristics:

- intelligent, but with very limited understanding of spoken English, no ability to read or write English, and no-one available to translate;
- extremely worried, tense and anxious about his medical condition and prognosis;
- low level of intelligence, barely literate, finds great difficulty in understanding and remembering instructions although he tries hard to be co-operative.

The *third person* takes the role of the observer, using the observer's checklist below.

Role-play the scene in which the health promoter is teaching the patient for ten minutes. The observer keeps time. Then give constructive feedback as follows:

- firstly, the 'health promoter' assesses herself, saying what she felt she did well, and identifying points she feels the need to work on in the future.
- secondly, the 'patient' describes how it felt to be the patient, identifying what the health promoter did or said which made him feel at ease/put down/ anxious/reassured/more confused, and so on.
- finally, the observer gives feedback using the checklist as a guide.

Communication checklist

1. Non-verbal aspects of communication
   eg. tone of voice, posture, gestures, facial expression, use of touch
2. Sequence and structure of key points
   eg. important things first, logical sequence, information in categories
3. Choice of language
   eg. appropriately simple and short, use of jargon/idioms, medical terms
4. Two-way communication
   eg. encourage patient to talk and express feelings, get feedback about how much is understood, open/closed/biased/multiple questions
5. Amount of information
   eg. too much or too little
6. Clarity of objective(s)
7. Use of repetition
8. Use of emphasis to stress important points
9. Any assumptions made but not checked
   eg. about previous knowledge, facilities for carrying out instructions, willingness to comply
10. Anything else?

Notes, References and Further Reading

1 For further reading on teaching and learning, in the context of health education in schools, see:

David K & Williams T (eds) (1987) *Health Education in Schools*. London: Harper & Row

Tones B K (1988) The role of the school in health promotion: the primacy of personal and social education. *Westminster Studies in Education*, **11**, 27–45

Williams D T & Roberts J (1985) *TEP Survey Report: Health Education in Schools and Teacher Education Institutions*. Health Education Unit, Southampton University

Williams T (1986) School health education 15 years on. *Health Education Journal*, **45**(1), 3–7

Reid D & Massey D (1986) Can school health education be more effective? *Health Education Journal*, **45**, 7–13

Anderson J (1986) Health skills: the power to choose. *Health Education Journal*, **45**(1), 19–24

Anderson J (1988) *HEA Health Skills Project: Training Manual*. Counselling and Career Development Unit, University of Leeds

Scottish Health Education Group (1986) *The Basic Curriculum Project*. Edinburgh: SHEG

Scottish Health Education Group/Scottish Consultative Council on the Curriculum (1989) *Promoting Good Health*. Edinburgh: SHEG/SCCC

For further reading on health education in the context of health care, see:

Scottish Health Education Group (1983) *Health Education In-Service Education and Training Needs of District Nurses, Health Visitors and Midwives*. Report of a Working Party of the Nursing Advisory Committee, Scottish Health Education Group, Edinburgh

Morris P (1988) Developing partnership with patients: the Cambridge communication skills project. In Weare K (ed.) *Developing Health Promotion in Undergraduate Medical Education*. London: Health Education Authority

For further reading on community-based health education, see:

Scottish Health Eduction Co-ordinating Committee (1984) *Health Education in Areas of Multiple Deprivation*. Edinburgh: Scottish Health Education Co-ordinating Group

Open University (1986) *A Review of Collaborative Health Education Programmes 1976–86*. Milton Keynes: Open University

Phillipson C & Strang P (1986) *Training and Education for an Ageing Society: New Perspectives for the Health and Social Services*. Working Papers on the Health of Older People No 3, Department of Adult and Continuing Education, University of Keele

For further reading on health education in the workplace, see:

McEwan J (1987) Health and work. In: *Health Education: Perspectives and Choices* (ed Sutherland I) Cambridge: National Extension College

Matheson H (ed) (1987) *Health Promotion in the Workplace.* Edinburgh: SHEG

For help with selecting the best way to give instructions and how to give instructions, see:

National Examination Board for Supervisory Management, Super Series, Open Learning module No. 304, *Giving Orders and Instructions.* Available from: Pergamon Open Learning, Headington Hill Hall, Oxford OX3 OBW. Telephone: 0865 64881

2 One study found that the use of this technique improved patients' recall by 17%:

Ley P *et al* (1973) A method for increasing patients' recall of information presented by doctors. *Psychological Medicine*, **3**, 217–220

3 For further reading on giving talks, see:

Kirkpatrick A L (1983) *The Complete Public Speaker's Manual.* London: Thorsons

Scott W (1984) *The Skills of Communicating.* Aldershot: Gower

For further reading on adult learning, see:

Brookfield S (1983) *Adult Learners, Adult Education and the Community.* Milton Keynes: Open University Press

Rogers A (1986) *Teaching Adults.* Milton Keynes: Open University Press

4 For an excellent summary of research into patient education, see:

Ley P (1988) *Communicating with patients—improving communication, satisfaction and compliance.* London: Croom Helm

See also:

Tones K, Tilford S & Robinson Y (1990) *Health Education—Effectiveness and Efficiency.* London: Chapman & Hall, Ch 5

5 This section is based on:

Ewles L & Shipster P (1981) *One-to-One Health Education.* East Sussex Area Health Authority, and

Ley P (1988) *Communicating with Patients—Improving Communication, Satisfaction and Compliance.* London: Croom Helm

6 For information about tape-recording and analysing an interview with a patient, see:

Perkins E R & Anderson D C (1981) *Self-assessment in the National Health Service.* London: Nafferton Books

7 For further study on patient education, see:

Distance Learning Centre, South Bank Polytechnic (1989) *Teaching Patients and Clients*. Managing Care Pack 9. London: South Bank Polytechnic

Ley P (1988) *Communicating with Patients—Improving Communication, Satisfaction and Compliance*. London: Croom Helm

Tones K, Tilford S & Robinson Y (1990) *Health Education—Effectiveness and Efficiency*. London: Chapman & Hall, Ch 5

Bartlett E (1985) Forum: patient education: eight principles from patient education research. *Preventive Medicine*, **14**, 667–9

Green C (1987) What can patient educators learn from 10 years of compliance research? *Patient Education and Counselling*, **10**, 167–74

Chapter 12 Working with Communities

Summary

This chapter is introduced with an explanation of the term 'community-based work in health promotion' and the range of activities it may include. Some key terms and principles are discussed, before looking at three particular ways of working with communities: community participation, community development and community health projects. Each of these includes an exercise, and there is also a case study of a community development project. The chapter ends by looking at the competences health promoters need to develop when working with communities.

As we have discussed many times in previous chapters, health promotion is the process of enabling people to increase control over, and improve, their health.[1] The challenge this presents is never more apparent than when considering people in the community who may be disadvantaged and discriminated against, and who feel powerless to do anything about their health. This chapter is about taking up that challenge, and working in the community with groups of people in a way which *does* enable them to take more control over their health.

Community-based Work in Health Promotion

By 'community-based work in health promotion' we mean work which directly involves the health promoter in working with groups of the public in a sustained way which will enable them to increase control over, and improve, their health. It involves different kinds of activities, possibly including:

- community development work;
- setting up a group and working with it on health issues;
- working on projects or campaigns focusing on a particular health issue (such as sickle

cell disease or drug addiction);
- providing health information services (such as well-woman information centres);
- health-related work undertaken by organisations with wider remits (such as health courses for older people run by national older people's organisations);
- advocacy projects (such as organisations undertaking interpreting and/or advocacy for Asian women);
- self-help groups getting together for mutual support on health problems.[2]

While this list begins to identify specific tasks that health promoters may find themselves having to tackle, it is necessary first to clarify some of the key terms and principles involved in community-based work.

Key Terms

Community. A community may be thought of as a network of people. The link between them may be where they live (such as a housing estate or neighbourhood), the work they do (such as 'the mining community'), their ethnic background (such as 'the Asian community') or other factors they have in common. The people in the network come together on the basis of a shared experience or concern, and identify for themselves which communities they feel they belong to. Networks may be formal or informal.

Community work. This means working with community groups and organisations to overcome the community's problems and improve their conditions of life. Community work aims to enhance the sense of solidarity and competence in the community. A *community worker* is usually a paid worker undertaking community work.

Community health work. This is community work with a focus on health concerns, but generally health is defined very broadly to include social and economic aspects, so that community health work may encompass almost as broad a range of activities as community work without a specific health remit.

Community action. This means activity carried out by people under their own control in order to improve their collective conditions. It may involve campaigning, negotiating with or challenging authorities and those with power.

Community participation. This is about involving the community in health work which is led by someone outside the community, for example, a worker employed by a statutory agency. The degree of participation may vary enormously.

Community development. This means working to stimulate and encourage communities to express their needs and to support them in their collective action. It is not about dealing with people's problems on a one-to-one basis; rather, it aims to develop the potential of a community. A *community development approach to health* involves working with groups of people to identify their own health concerns, and to take appropriate action. *Community development health workers* are essentially facilitators, locally based, whose role is to help people in the community to acquire the skills, knowledge and confidence to act on health issues. They are usually community workers by background, rather than health professionals.

Community health projects. This is a loose term applied to programmes of work which are organised by agencies for the improvement of health in a community, or to local organisations aiming to improve health by supporting some combination of community activity, self-help, community action and/or community development.[3]

Finally, it is worth mentioning that in the health service the word *community* is often used as an adjective to describe anything that is not based in hospital; examples are 'community care', 'community nurses', 'community services' and 'the Community Unit'.

Community participation, community development and community health projects will be explored in greater depth later in the chapter, but first we look at some principles of community health work.

Principles of Community-based Work

We identify four key principles, as follows.

The Centrality of the Community

It is the *community* which defines its own needs, not the health workers. Community-based work is essentially a '*bottom-up*' process, rather than a 'top-down' process where those with power and authority make the decisions. Community workers recognise and value the health experience and knowledge that exists in the community, and seek to use it for everyone's benefit.

The Facilitator Role of the Community Health Worker

Community health workers do not perceive themselves as 'experts' in health, but as facilitators whose role is to validate, encourage and empower people to define their own health needs and to meet them. They start where the community is, recognising and valuing people's own abilities and experiences. They involve people in the community health work from the very beginning, encouraging and supporting them in working together. Knowledge and skills are shared and demystified. Community health workers aim to complement as well as challenge the statutory services by making people's access to statutory agencies easier, and making the agencies more accountable to the people they serve.

The Importance of Addressing Inequalities

A central concern in community-based health work is the need to challenge and change the many forms of disadvantage, oppression and discrimination which people face, and which adversely affect their health. There is acute awareness of the need to address inequalities in health and health services and to focus on the social, environmental and economic determinants of health.

Work therefore focuses particularly on the needs of disadvantaged and oppressed groups, which is why work with women and minority ethnic and black groups is prominent. A central way of working is to bring people in such groups together for support and information-sharing, and to enable them to bring about change through collective action. There is no denying that the work is political, because it means working towards greater equality and social justice. It means working with people who experience powerlessness and inequality as part of their everyday lives, and working towards a redistribution of resources and power.

A Broad Perspective on Health

Health is perceived broadly and holistically as positive well-being, including social, emotional, mental and societal aspects as well as physical ones. It is not seen merely as the absence of disease, and is not limited by medical or epidemiological views of what constitutes a health problem or issue. Health is seen to be affected by social, environmental, economic and political factors.

Community Participation

Participation is a word that is used very widely to mean a range of activities, from those that are merely tokenistic to those which are firmly rooted in the concept of empowerment. We look at two aspects where you may be involved: first, in planning new developments, and then by identifying practical ways of supporting the principle of community participation.

Community Participation in Planning

The amount of community participation in planning health work organised by an agency (such as a health or local authority) can vary along a spectrum of none to high, as follows:[4]

No participation: the community is told nothing, and is not involved in any way.

Very low participation—the community is informed: the agency makes a plan and announces it. The community is convened or notified in other ways in order to be informed; compliance is expected.

Low participation—the community is offered 'token' consultation: the agency tries to promote a plan and seeks support or at least sufficient sanction so that the plan can go ahead. It is unwilling to modify the plan unless absolutely necessary.

Moderate participation—the community advises through a consultation

process: the agency presents a plan and invites questions, comments and recommendations. It is prepared to modify the play.

High participation—the community plan jointly: representatives of the agency and the community sit down together from the beginning to devise a plan.

Very high participation—the community has delegated authority: the agency identifies and presents an issue to the community, defines the limits and asks the community to make a series of decisions which can be embodied in a plan which it will accept.

Highest participation—the community has control: the agency asks the community to identify the issue and make all the key decisions about goals and plans. It is willing to help the community at each step to accomplish its goals, even to the extent of delegating administrative control of the work.

Health promoters involved in planning initiatives in the community can use this framework to consider the extent to which their agencies invite communities to participate.

Ways of Developing Community Participation

Community participation can be encouraged and supported in many ways at different levels. We suggest some ways in which you may be able to develop community participation, particularly if you work for a statutory agency:[5]

Be open about policies and plans. Publicise your policies, invite comments and recommendations on your plans, involve representatives on planning and management groups.

Plan for the community's expressed needs. When planning services, help the community to express its own needs as it sees them, and take this into account when planning services.

Decentralise planning. Set up planning and management of health and allied services on a neighbourhood basis, encouraging and enabling the public's involvement.

Develop joint forums. Develop joint forums, such as patient participation groups in doctors' practices, where lay people and professionals can work together in partnership.

Develop networks. Encourage individuals or groups to come together, thus increasing their collective knowledge and power to change things.

Provide support, advice and training for community groups. Provide opportunities for lay people to develop their knowledge, confidence and skills, such as in running groups, speaking in public, or finding their way around bureaucratic statutory organisations. This could be provided through informal discussions, perhaps on a 'drop in' basis, or structured training courses.

Provide information. Provide information about health issues, details of useful local and national organisations, leaflets, posters and books.

Provide help with funding and resources. Help local groups to obtain funding from statutory agencies, and provide other sorts of practical help such as a place to meet or facilities to photocopy materials.

Support advocacy projects. Support projects which enable people who are otherwise excluded from the community to have a voice, such as interpreting/advocacy schemes for Asian patients.

Exercise—Developing community participation in your work

Consider the following list of ways in which you can encourage community participation in working for health:

- Be open about policies and plans
- Plan for the community's expressed needs
- Decentralise planning
- Develop joint forums
- Develop networks
- Provide support, advice and training for community groups
- Provide information
- Provide help with funding and resources
- Support advocacy projects

(If you are not sure what is meant by these, look back at the explanations above.)

To what extent do you think these things are desirable?

To what extent do you do these things already?

From this list, can you identify ways in which you would like to increase community participation in your work?

Can you identify any other ways in which you would like to increase community participation in your work?

Given that there may be some obstacles to doing what you would ideally like to do, can you identify a practical way forward for acting on at least one of the things you would like to do?

Work either individually, in pairs or small groups.

Community Development

However much you might seek people's participation, it may be that they feel so alienated, dissatisfied or generally unwanted that participation is the last thing they wish to do. In this situation it is necessary to develop a climate and culture where participation can happen. You need to encourage, enable and support people, and *community development* is a way of doing this.

Community development is much more than community *participation*. It means working with people to identify their *own* health concerns, and to support and facilitate them in their collective action. It means adhering firmly to the principles of community-based work we have outlined above, with the community development worker having the role of a facilitator.

The exercise 'Thinking about Community Development' is designed to help you to consider what community development work means in practice.

Exercise—Thinking about community development[6]

Working individually, or in pairs or small groups, work through the following questionnaire. If you are working with other people, discuss the reasons for the answers you give. You do not have to reach a consensus—after you have listened to each other's views, you can agree to disagree.

Tick whether you think each of the following statements is true or false:

Community development is about:	True	False
1. Fostering a sense of community among people	____	____
2. Helping people to see the root causes of their ill-health	____	____
3. Enabling a statutory authority to show that it 'cares'	____	____
4. Getting involved in a political process	____	____
5. Doing away with 'experts' and 'professionals'	____	____
6. Confronting forms of discrimination such as racism and sexism	____	____
7. Saving money on services by helping people to help themselves	____	____
8. Promoting equal access to resources such as health services	____	____
9. Enabling a community worker to become a leader/spokesperson for the community	____	____
10. Helping people to develop confidence and become more articulate about their needs	____	____
11. Campaigning for a better environment such as improved housing, transport and play facilities	____	____
12. Controlling social unrest, e.g by providing activities for bored youth	____	____
13. Helping working class people become more like middle class people in terms of their attitudes and behaviour	____	____

continued on next page

continued

14. Recognising and valuing the skills, knowledge and expertise of individuals and groups in the community ____ ____
15. Beginning a process of redistributing wealth, power and resources ____ ____

Now add any other points you think community development is, or is not, about:

____

____

____

____

____

____

The following case study illustrates community development in practice, demonstrating how the community and the community's own expressed needs were central to the development, the workers acted as facilitators, inequalities in health were addressed and a broad perspective on health was taken. It also shows how local people were empowered to take action.

Case study—Community development in practice—The Granton Community Health Project[7]

A pilot project was funded in Granton, Scotland, to raise awareness of health issues in a deprived area and to find ways whereby people in the community could communicate their health needs and concerns. The project was staffed by a community development worker and a health visitor, with a research worker coming in at a later date.

The community development worker started by getting to know and documenting all the local resources provided by statutory and voluntary agencies in the area as well as community-based groups. A small survey of local residents and professionals was then carried out to provide information on concepts of health, health needs and so on, and this highlighted interesting differences in the views of residents and professionals.

To encourage local people to give their opinions and become more involved, a larger survey was planned with suggestions from the residents. Eighteen local people were trained and paid as interviewers. The survey helped to build up a picture of health needs in the area, but it was also part of a process of education for the interviewers themselves, who were found to have improved self-image and a raised awareness of conditions in the area. Their desire to discuss some of the issues in greater depth led to setting up a group which then drew in more residents by personal contact. Several groups were initiated in the same way, as people came up with problems and issues they wanted to address. These groups were gradually taken over and run by local residents as they gained confidence.

continued on next page

continued

Some groups remained small and short-lived, but others had far-reaching effects. One example was a women's health discussion group, which started by looking at topics such as stress, childbirth and talking to doctors, and then focused on the problem of damp housing. The group prepared a tape-slide presentation showing the problem and how it affected their lives. This was shown at a seminar at Edinburgh University, and stimulated a research project to investigate the effects of damp housing on health. The process of putting forward their concerns helped group members to gain confidence and demonstrated that residents from a deprived area could stimulate academic research on their own chosen priorities.

Other long-term outcomes included a tranquilliser support group, a drop-in stress centre, and an elderly people's forum which secured funding for a minibus, an information worker on pensioners' issues and a visiting scheme for frail elderly people.

The evaluation of the project by the University of Aberdeen concluded that it had been successful in meeting most of its objectives. It had opened up channels of communication between professionals and residents, it had developed ways of fostering the skills of some of the residents in dealing with health issues and had shown how some of these issues could be tackled by lay people in new ways.

Some Implications of the Community Development Approach

If you choose to adopt a community development approach, it is important to understand the implications. The experience of community development projects around the country has shown that five areas of tension are likely to surface.[8] We identify these below, and some ways of trying to prevent them.

Different priorities: priorities chosen by communities may not be the same as those of local statutory agencies or indeed the body who is funding the work. A common difference is that health problems as defined by health workers are likely to be about physical health problems, risk factors for major illnesses and low uptake of health services, such as low birth-weight babies, heavy drinking and poor immunisation rates. Community priorities, on the other hand, are often about social conditions, such as housing, poor child care provision and lack of good public transport, and this must be clearly understood and accepted at the outset of any community development work.

A threat to local health workers: if local people gain confidence and become more articulate through the process of community development, they are likely to voice concern and criticism about local health services. Furthermore, the prospect of members of the community taking an active role in policy-making and planning may be alien to many managers and field-workers in statutory agencies. A thorough educational grounding in the rationale and principles of community-based work is required, although setting this up and getting people to listen may in itself be a daunting task.

No instant results: community development work is slow; it takes time to get to know a community and to build up trust with local people. It may be *years* before there is any tangible outcome. Projects with short-term funding are therefore likely to be expected to work in unrealistic time-scales, and are likely to fail if quick results are expected. Secure funding for several years, with realistic objectives, is fundamental to success.

A token gesture or an easy option: well-meaning authorities who want to 'do something' (or be seen to be doing something) about inequalities in health may set up a community health project as a way of addressing the issue. Clearly it cannot be 'the answer' to complex and deeply-rooted causes of poor health; at best it can make a valuable contribution, but at worst it can divert attention from the real political solutions to the problems.

Evaluation conflicts: outside agencies may expect to see results in terms of traditional 'outcomes' such as improved immunisation rates, a measurable change in community behaviour (less drunkenness, for example) or lower rates of hospital admission. However, the objectives of a community development project are rarely couched in such terms, and are more likely to be concerned with far less easily measured results such as increased self-confidence, increased public participation in health planning or better communication between the community and statutory agencies. Once again, education in the process, principles, aims and likely outcomes are essential for all concerned.

Community Health Projects

We now turn from thinking about community development to considering how you might be involved in a *community health project*. (This was defined at the beginning of the chapter as a programme of work organised by an agency or a local organisation with the aim of improving health by some combination of community activity, self-help, community action and/or community development.) For example, you might want to set up a project to work with young parents on a housing estate with the aim of improving their confidence, skills and mutual support in parenting, or with older people in a particular area to encourage social activities with a health benefit, such as relaxation and exercise groups, tea dances or lunch clubs.

In order to think systematically about setting up and running a community health project, we suggest using the *Planning and evaluation flowchart* from Chapter Six. Additional help can be gained from reading the growing number of community health projects that have been written up so that the processes, successes and failures, and lessons learnt, can be shared.[9]

The experience of community health workers has highlighted specific issues which it is helpful to consider. These points are discussed below, set out within the *Planning and evaluation* framework.[10] This is *not* a comprehensive guide to setting up and running community health projects; it is intended to complement the information in Chapter Six, and identify points which are especially relevant to community health project work.

Stage 1: Identifying Needs and Priorities

At this stage, two particular issues are: how do you get to know the community and who do you consult?

Getting to know the community and its needs: get all the relevant information you can about the health of the community. Search out data from the health authority and local authority.

Try contacting neighbourhood centres, community groups, voluntary organisations and tenants associations. People who might be able to put you in touch with these include local workers in health and social services, local churches and schools, the local Council for Voluntary Service, the Community Health Council and the local Council for Racial Equality. Talk to members of the public, perhaps at local markets and festivals. It might be useful to hold public meetings or conduct a small survey.

Talk to local professionals, but bear in mind that professional perceptions will often stem from a problem-centred view of a locality; for example, police will talk about crime, social workers about the numbers of children on the 'at-risk' register.

Local newspapers may be a useful source of information about the needs, interests and activities of a locality, and may even have a library service which will select material on a particular issue for you.

Another approach is to *walk*—not drive—around the neighbourhood. Groups of young people on street corners, smells from fast-food shops, and the range and price of goods in shop windows can reveal a lot about local life-style and socioeconomic conditions.

Consulting before setting up: consult with local health and social service workers at a very early stage. Consult with the community only if you are sure the project is going to happen: consultation before funding is secure, for example, could raise people's expectations falsely, waste their time and diminish their trust.

Stages 2 and 3: Setting Aims and Objectives, and Deciding the Best Way of Achieving Them

Key issues here are about being flexible and realistic. It is helpful to *consult* the people you have already made contact with, and the management group/steering group of the project (if there is one). These people may help you to set realistic, achievable aims and objectives, and to work out the best means of achieving them.

Flexibility is vital because community work is essentially a developmental process, so you need to review and modify your objectives regularly. Objectives may change, and indeed should change, if new opportunities arise and/or previous objectives no longer seem achievable or compatible with changing needs.

Being realistic: this applies to identifying *what* you plan to achieve, and *by when*. For example, if you are planning a community development approach, ensure that you have a realistic timescale; three years is suggested as a reasonable minimum.

Stage 4: Identifying Resources

People and **premises** are two key resources.

People: by bringing people with a common interest or experience together, you may find that the collective energy of the group generates ideas for future action and you can begin to share the work. This means that your role may also begin to change, from being an initiator to being a supporter.

It is also important to think about the training and development needs of the people who are the key resource of the project. Not only project workers, but also the project management committee (if there is one) and local health professionals may need help in understanding what this type of work is all about. What training is needed, who will do it and how will it be funded?

Premises: you need to consider what premises you need: rooms for meeting in (large and small meetings), a room for a crèche, a place to keep and use equipment such as video equipment and photocopiers, a library/place where people can look up information? Access for wheelchairs, pushchairs and prams? Running water and toilets? Facilities for making refreshments or meals? Good access by public transport? Well-lit premises so that people feel safe going there after dark?

You also need to consider the 'image' of possible premises: if you are offered space in a clinic, for example, this may mean that people perceive the project to be part of the statutory health services.

Stage 5: Planning Evaluation Methods

Bear in mind the possibility of evaluation conflicts, which we discussed in the previous section, and make sure that your evaluation looks at both process and outcome and identifies realistic ways of assessing what may be very small changes over long periods of time.

Stage 6: Setting an Action Plan

There are many things to consider here, but the main one is to identify what you plan to do step by achievable step. You may need to build the following activities into your action plan:

Reviewing aims and priorities: it is necessary to review continuously the aims and priorities originally set down for the project, and compare them with those of the people who are now involved. You may need to modify your original aims, and constantly check whose agenda you are working to—your own or the community's?

Consulting and being accountable to the community: we recommended consultation before you set up, but this needs to continue throughout the life of the project. Once established, you have a continuing responsibility to tell the community what the project's role is and what work is going on. This could be through meetings, newsletters and open days, for example.

Arranging a management committee or steering group: a management committee or steering group should provide a secure foundation for the project, taking responsibility for its continued development, its policies and management tasks such as fund raising and recruiting. It should also provide support for the workers. Usually the workers are members of the group; they should not be expected to run the management committee themselves, but sometimes this is the case—not a desirable practice because it leads to confusion about who is managing who and puts an unreasonable burden on the workers.

A management group could consist both of local workers such as health visitors and social workers, and local people, perhaps representing groups with whom the project is in contact. It may be helpful to get the members of a management/steering committee together for a day, to talk through the issues, clarify aims and foster a sense of teamwork.

Writing job descriptions: paid project workers need clear job descriptions, specifying what is included. For example, does the job include fund-raising, doing their own typing, servicing or even running the management committee meetings, keeping the accounts, evaluating, writing progress reports?

Ensuring support for the project workers: recognise the value of networking as a means of informal training and support. By 'networking' we mean making time and resources available to meet other people doing similar work and to link with other community health projects in different parts of the country. This enables information and ideas to be shared, problems to be discussed and encouragement given. It fosters a vital sense of not 'going it alone'. The need to ensure that project workers are not isolated in what may be very slow and, at times, discouraging work cannot be overstressed. Networking also means that more people will know about your project and you may get more support. Other people, too, may benefit if they have also been experiencing isolation.

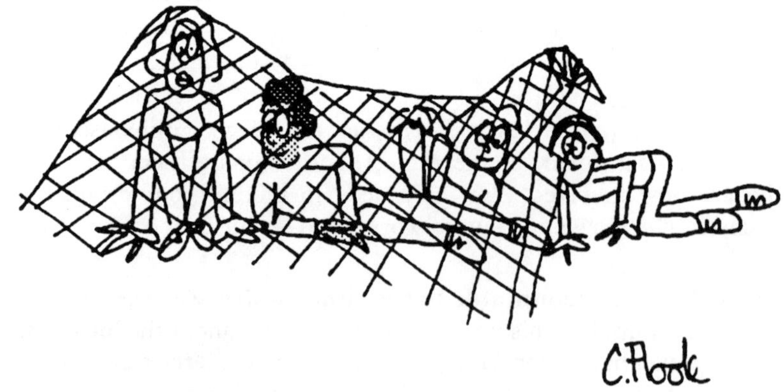

Networking fosters a vital sense of 'not going it alone

Formalising your project group: it may be helpful at some stage to look at the costs and benefits of formalising a project group which started off as a loose collection of interested people. The advantages of having a formal organisation are that it can apply for financial help and for recognition as a legitimate body; the disadvantages might be that control could be exercised from outside, or that members are attracted who turn out to be more of a hindrance than a help. The local Council for Voluntary Service can be extremely useful since it provides a helpful service for newly-formed groups, and affiliation to the Council brings credibility in itself.

Dealing with friends and enemies: the issues your project is concerned with will probably have a local history, and be likely to have both lost and won support in the past. You need to identify other interest groups, and decide how to tackle them. Study the tactics and arguments of any 'opposition' and plan your strategy.

Stage 7: Implementing your Plan

As you implement your plan, you may run into difficulties because of flagging interest, a feeling of losing your way, and, finally, that the project has to come to an end. Some suggestions about these three issues now follow.

Keeping going: with the passage of time, people may lose their enthusiasm. You may be able to provide additional impetus by having the advantage of being involved as a whole or part of your paid work. You need to be sensitive to the many ways by which a project can lose its way, and in such circumstances you may be able to help by:

- discovering what similar activities are taking place elsewhere and circulating details;
- drawing the issue to the attention of relevant statutory agencies, and conveying the response to the group;
- helping the group to produce their own health promotion materials such as posters, leaflets or even a video, and distributing them;
- looking at other health promotion material on topics of interest;
- encouraging members of the project to talk about their work to other people, such as groups of interested professionals and students;
- sending everyone a circular to remind them of meetings;
- providing practical support such as photocopying or typing;
- introducing new members.

Working out what to do next: if you feel that you have lost your way, it can help to write down what information you have found, what contacts you have made, what needs and aims you have identified and what you have done so far. Then seek the views of your management/steering group (if there is one) or the impartial views of someone who has not been involved. The exercise below *Planning community health work* may help to provide a focus for working out what to do next.

Leavings and endings: there comes a point when your involvement has to stop, maybe because you change your job or the priorities of your work, or because the project work has been taken on by local people. Occasionally, you may need to recognise that you have done all you can do, and there is no potential in the project any more. Ending your involvement provides the opportunity for a final evaluation of what has been achieved, what your own contribution has been and making recommendations for future action.

Exercise—Planning community health work

The following exercise may be useful when you are starting community health work or taking stock part way through a piece of work.

Complete the following statements as far as you can:

The key issue is . . .
The people I need to talk to are . . .
The documents I need to read are . . .
I can get to know more about the community by . . .
The information that is likely to be available is . . .
I intend to look for this information by . . .
Work done on this issue elsewhere is . . .
The people who are likely to be supportive are . . .
The people I should avoid offending are . . .
The period of time I can spend on this issue is . . .
The amount of time I can give it during this period is . . .
The person/people I will talk to in order to work out what to do next is/are . . .

Developing Competences in Community Work

To be a successful community health worker, you need to develop a range of knowledge and skills, and have certain crucial values and attitudes.[11]

In terms of *values and attitudes*, you will need to be committed to the principles and ideals of community-based work which we outlined earlier in this chapter: the centrality of the community, your own role as a facilitator rather than an 'expert', the importance of addressing inequalities and a broad perspective on health.

In order to hold these values and attitudes with depth and conviction, you will need *knowledge* of key issues, such as the extent and cause of inequalities in health, the effects of racism, sexism and other forms of oppression on health, and awareness of the structures, policies and powers which influence the lives and health of communities. You will also need to be clear about your own particular political ideologies.

Other areas of *knowledge* include knowledge of local health resources: who and where to go to for information, advice and materials on health issues, etc. Knowledge of local health services and social services is vital; so is understanding how local statutory and voluntary agencies work, and how to use 'the system' effectively. An understanding of the community itself is of course vital too. (See the section above *Getting to know the community and its needs*.)

A range of *skills* is required. It is important to have the skills of raising awareness of inequalities and discrimination, and being able to counter these by taking positive action when appropriate and working in an anti-discriminatory way.

Other skills are to do with working with people: being able to communicate well, facilitate groups and have effective meetings, for example. You also need the skills of planning and management, using and producing health promotion materials, and working for political change. (All of these are discussed in more detail in other chapters.)

A list of some useful resources is given in the Notes which follow.[12]

Notes, References and Further Reading

1 Definition in:

World Health Organisation (1984) Health Promotion: a WHO Discussion Document on the Concepts and Principles. Reprinted in: *Journal of the Institute of Health Education*, **23**(1), 1985. For discussion of this definition, see Chapter Two.

2 London Community Health Resource & National Council for Voluntary Organisations (1987) *Guide to Community Health Projects*. London: National Community Health Resource

3 These definitions draw on the work of:

Channon G. In Adams L & Smithies J (1990) *Community Participation and Health Promotion*. London: Health Education Authority

The definition of community development also draws on:

Association of Metropolitan Authorities (1989) *Community Development, the Local Authority Role*. London: Association of Metropolitan Authorities

4 This framework is adapted from:

Brager & Sprecht (1973) *Community Organising*. Columbia University Press

5 These suggestions are adapted from:

Adams L & Smithies J (1990) *Community Participation and Health Promotion*. London: Health Education Authority

6 Adapted from a questionnaire by Lee Adams and David Hawkins and reproduced by their kind permission.

7 This account is taken from:

Whitehead M (1989) *Swimming Upstream: Trends and Prospects in Education for Health*. London: King's Fund Institute

Whitehead's summary refers to a fuller account in:

Research Unit in Health and Behavioural Change, University of Edinburgh (1989) *Changing the Public Health*. Chichester: Wiley, Ch 8, Jones J Promoting health through community development

The Granton Community Health Project can also be contacted directly at: The Health Hut, 3 West Pilton Park, Edinburgh EH4 4EC

See also:

Hunt S (1989) *Community Development and Health Promotion in a Deprived Area: Final Report*. Working Paper. Edinburgh: Research Unit in Health and Behavioural Change

Drummond N (1989) Evaluation of a community health project: the experience from West Granton, Edinburgh. In Martin C & McQueen D (eds) *Readings for a New Public Health*. Edinburgh University Press

8 Whitehead M (1989) *Swimming Upstream: Trends and Prospects in Education for Health*. London: King's Fund Institute, p 34

9 Community Projects Foundation (1988) *Action for Health*. London: Community Projects Foundation, Health Education Authority & Scottish Health Education Group

Community Health Initiatives Resource Unit & London Community Health Resource (1987) *Guide to Community Health Projects*. London: National Community Health Resource

Ellis J (1989) *Breaking New Ground: Community Development with Asian Communities*. London: Bedford Square Press, in association with the Community Projects Foundation

Kenner C (1986) *Whose Needs Count? Community Action for Health*. London: Bedford Square Press/National Council for Voluntary Organisations

10 This section draws extensively on material in:

'Guidelines for setting up projects' in Community Health Initiatives Resource Unit & London Community Health Resource (1987) *Guide to Community Health Projects*, Ch 4. London: National Community Health Resource. Readers are recommended to read this guide for fuller details, and

Henderson P & Thomas D N (1980) *Skills in Neighbourhood Work*, National Institute of Social Services Library, no. 39. London: Allen & Unwin.

Also see:

Perkins E (1988) *Working with the Wider Community: a Handbook for Managers and Trainers*. Nottingham Health Education & Promotion Unit, Memorial House, Standard Hill, Nottingham NG1 6FX

11 This section is derived from:

Smithies J (1987) *Training Needs of Community Health Workers*. National Community Health Resource, unpublished report on community health workers training project.

12 Useful agencies are:

National Community Health Resource (NCHR), 15 Britannia Street, London WC1X 9JP. Telephone: 071-837 2426. This organisation provides information, training and support to community health initiatives, publishes a quarterly newsletter *Community Health Action*, and directories, guides, reports, books and teaching materials.

The following NCHR publications are especially recommended for health promoters embarking on community-based work:

Guide to Community Health Projects (1987)
Grassle L & Kingsley S (1986) *Measuring Change, Making Changes: an Approach to Evaluation*
McNaught A (1987) *Health Action and Ethnic Minorities.* London: NCHR/ Bedford Square Press

Federation of Community Work Training Groups, 356 Glossop Road, Sheffield S10 2HW. Telephone: 0742 739391. This is a federation of twelve regional training groups, funded by the Home Office but with the emphasis on regional development of local training for people working voluntarily or paid within their own communities.

Standing Conference for Community Development (SCCD), 356 Glossop Road, Sheffield S10 2HW. Telephone: 0742 701718. This is a group of regional and national representatives from organisations whose work involves community development.

Chapter 13
Changing Policy and Practice

Summary

This chapter begins with a consideration of who makes health policy changes and continues by discussing how health promoters can challenge health-damaging policies. Sections on understanding the characteristics of power and influence and the politics of influence follow, illustrated with a case study. This is followed by sections on developing and implementing policies, a case study exercise on policy implementation, and a section on campaigning. The chapter concludes with a discussion on how to implement changes successfully.

Health promoters are in the business of influencing policies and practices which affect health. (By 'policies' we mean broad plans of action, which set the direction for detailed planning.) These can be at any level, from national (such as policies set by government or political parties about, for example, housing, transport and future directions for the NHS) to the level of day-to-day work of a health promoter (such as what sort of health promotion clinics will be run in a GP practice, or what resources will be devoted to specific health promotion activities in an environmental health department).

In order to influence policy and practice, you need to understand how power is distributed and exercised between people at any level, from a group of colleagues to those in positions of great authority or influence. You need to be able to use that knowledge to affect decisions. (This process of understanding the distribution of power and how it is used, and using that knowledge to further your work, is what we mean by 'being political'.)

Changing policy and practice includes working with statutory, voluntary and commercial organisations to influence them to develop health-promoting policies for their staff and to produce health-enhancing products and services. It also includes working for healthy public policies and economic and regulatory changes requiring campaigning, lobbying and taking political action.

In this chapter, we look first at who makes health policies and the contribution of health promoters to making and changing policies. We then focus on four practical aspects of changing policy and practice, which we see as especially relevant in health promotion: understanding the politics of influence, developing and implementing health promotion policies, campaigning and implementing changes successfully.

Who Makes Health Policies?

The importance of making policy changes as an integral part of health promotion is increasingly recognised. We are concerned here with both *local* policies and *national* policies, because health promoters working at a local level can press for the introduction of policies at both levels and have an influence on how they are implemented. Furthermore, the development of local policies cannot be divorced from government policies. The nature of, and the resources for, health service, local authority and voluntary organisation work are shaped by central government's policy and by the allocation of funds. The evolution of national policy is, in turn, influenced by representations from health and local authorities and voluntary agencies.

At a local level, many policies and priorities are now jointly agreed, and this can improve their effectiveness.[1] For example, policies can be agreed by the Local Authority, the District Health Authority, the Family Health Services Authority, and other relevant community organisations such as the Council for Racial Equality, trade unions, housing associations and voluntary organisations. Another innovation is that some local authorities are undertaking health and/or environmental audits of their services. This involves examining the impact on health and/or the environment of all current and planned activities of each department of the local authority. The purpose is to develop practical ways in which the current health and environmental impact of services could be improved and to inform the development of a corporate approach to new health and environmental policies.

Until 1991, there was no formal national policy for implementing the World Health Organisation's (WHO) *Health For All* strategy. The UK Government was strongly of the view that precisely targeted local initiatives, with which local communities can identify, were the most appropriate way forward for Britain.[2] Nevertheless, many national bodies and groups were, and continue to be, active in reviewing policies at national level and across the country, and in making recommendations for the future.[3]

However, in 1991 the UK government published a consultative document which outlined a strategy for improving health in England, with comparable strategies for Wales, Scotland and Northern Ireland expected to follow.[4] This picked up on the need for national policies and programmes on health, as the WHO Health For All strategy had proposed. It emphasised the need to focus on priority health problems, concentrate on health promotion and disease prevention as much as on treatment, and encourage co-operation between different agencies at national and local level. It identified priority areas for action (such as preventing heart disease) and suggested clear objectives and targets, with key roles at national and local level for a wide range of agencies, including Government Departments, the NHS, local government, industry and commerce and the voluntary sector. Following consultation, it is expected that a finalised national strategy for health will be produced, which is generally considered to be a significant and welcome development.

Challenging Health-damaging Policy[5]

There are two aspects to changing policies and practice: changing an existing policy, and developing new policies. Later in this chapter we turn to how you can develop new policies, but first we look at a question which health promoters often pose: what can you do when you are faced with policies which you perceive as health damaging?

This question often induces feelings of helplessness and frustration because such policies come from 'high places' such as national government or (closer to home) your own employing authority or even your own direct manager. To protest may seem a futile waste of energy and can cause a conflict of loyalty between wanting to press for what you see as right and what is decreed to be right by your employing authority. To protest or take action may be seen as troublemaking or too political.

There is no easy answer to this issue, but there are some positive steps worth considering.

Use your vote. At the next general or local election, look at the health implications in the policy manifestos. Raise questions about healthy policy with doorstep canvassers, at public meetings and by writing to candidates. All this can be done in your capacity as a private citizen rather than a health worker.

Use your professional association or trade union. These groups can raise issues at a national and local level, and can be a powerful voice. You can play your part by joining and supporting their activities, and raising the issues you feel strongly about.

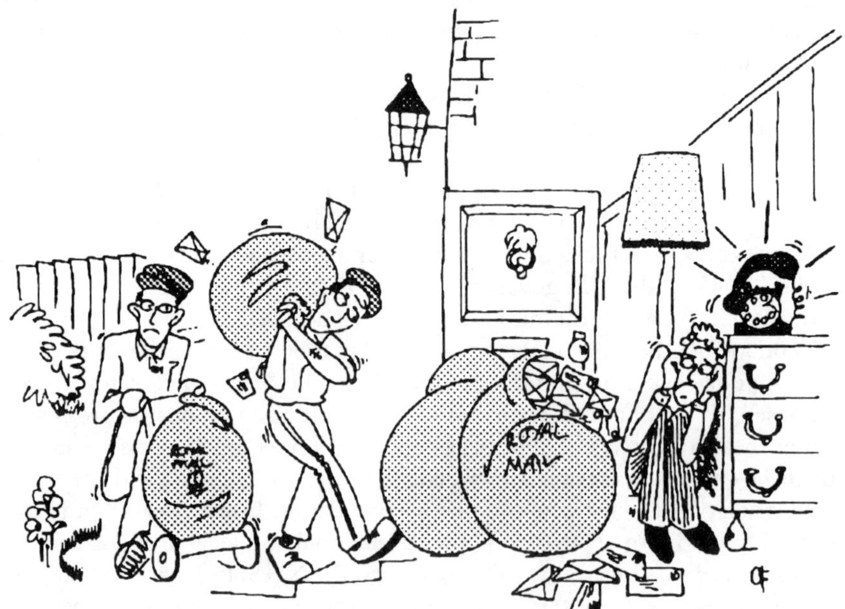

Lobby your MP

Use your representative. There are many people whose job it is to represent your interests. At national level, it is your MP. So if you want to raise an issue at national level, lobby your MP: send letters, telephone, attend 'surgeries'. At local level, do the same with your local councillor.[6] You can also contact your professional association or union local branch representative.

Use your collective power. If you are concerned about an issue at your place of work, it may help to find out if colleagues feel the same about it. If they do, join together so that you raise the issue collectively, which is likely to give it more impact and take the heat off any one individual.

However, many areas of policy development are not controversial and, indeed, can be a positive and rewarding part of the day-to-day work of health promoters. The main thrust is likely to be in developing, changing and implementing local policies. To do this you need to understand the characteristics of power and influence and to be competent at exerting influence, when necessary. We look at this in the next sections.

Characteristics of Power and Influence[7]

Power is the ability to influence others. There are four generally recognised types of power which are relevant to health promotion work:

Position power is the power vested in someone because of their position in an organisation. For example, the chief executive of a local authority has position power.

Resource power is the power to allocate, or limit, resources, including money and staff. It often goes hand-in-hand with position power. For example, a general manager in the Health Service has both position power and the power to regulate the use of resources. If you have the power to control the allocation of any resources that people want, then you have a real source of power. Every health promoter will have some power because there will be people who want the skills or services on offer.

Expert power is power related to special expertise. A consultant in the Health Service will have the expert power associated with his clinical specialty.

Personal power is the power that comes from the personal attributes of a person—including strong personality, charisma and ability to inspire. It is closely related to leadership qualities, such as above average intelligence, initiative, self-confidence and the ability to rise above a situation and see it in perspective (the 'helicopter' trait). However, effective leaders are not always charismatic, and what makes a leader effective in one situation may cause him to be less effective in changed circumstances. The classic example of this is Sir Winston Churchill: the attributes which made him effective in wartime were not so appropriate in peacetime.

You may sometimes be in the position of wishing to exert influence on people who have a stronger power base—for example, a health visitor may wish to influence a general practitioner to adopt a policy of supporting the running of antenatal clinics in the local minority ethnic group's community centre. Or a community worker may want to lobby local councillors about the need for more recreational facilities for young people on a housing estate. To do this requires skills in influencing.

Before embarking on an attempt to influence someone who is more powerful, first consider (as always) the basic questions in the planning process, such as: What are your aims? What resources do you need? Is the investment going to be worth it? Could the aim be achieved more easily another way? (See Chapter Six *Planning and Evaluating*.)

The Politics of Influence[8]

The elements of any strategy aiming to change policy and practice could include:

- key aspects of planning
- making allies
- networking
- making deals

We now consider each of these in turn.

Planning

Three particular aspects of planning are useful to consider: undertaking a force field analysis, identifying stakeholders and considering your timing.

Undertake a force field analysis. A force field analysis identifies the helping and hindering forces in your situation and helps to pinpoint how you can influence the process to make progress towards change. You identify how you can increase the power of the helping forces and decrease the power of the hindering forces. (There is an example of a force field analysis in the Exercise *What helps and hinders your health promotion work* at the end of Chapter Four.)

Identify the stakeholders. The stakeholders are those people with a vested interest in the issue, who wish to influence what is done and how it is done. They are obviously powerful forces in the situation. It may be difficult to identify all the stakeholders, because some of them may not wish to be visible and try to work covertly through others.

Time your action. It is also important to consider when to introduce a proposal or when to delay. If people are already preoccupied with major issues, now may not be the right moment to make a new proposal. On the other hand, if a proposal will help other people to attain their own objectives, now may be a good time.

Making Allies

Identify which of the stakeholders could be allies, and gain their trust and confidence in order to establish and maintain an alliance. It helps to pay attention to their concerns, values, beliefs and behaviour patterns, and see what you need to do in order to form an effective working alliance.

For example, if you are concerned about the way in which HIV positive people may be treated in an organisation, you might identify a personnel officer as a key stakeholder. So find out: Is she concerned about it? Does she think it is important for her organisation? What kind of way does she work: is she likely to respond best to a lively discussion on the subject or to a well-argued paper on the need for policy, backed up with facts and figures? Does she like time to make decisions? Will she be happy to leave you to take the lead, or will she want to feel that the initiative lies with her?[9]

Networking

Many people working in organisations belong to one or more interest groups which meet to discuss, debate and exchange information on issues that concern the members. These interest groups are *networks*. By playing an active role in networks, people can extend their influence. Networks provide access to information to help with making a case, to people with experience of successful influencing, and to other resources. There are different types of networks:

Professional networks—members of the same profession. Professional networks may attempt to influence employers and organisations to reconsider their policies or to develop new policies for the future. Professional networks institute criteria for professional practice and are active in the professional development of their members.

Elitist networks—members of an elitist group who can join by invitation only. The network operates by personal contact and personal introduction, such as 'old boy' links. Members of such networks may have considerable power and influence, often through their position in organisations.

Pressure groups—members wish to pursue certain objectives which may be environmental, social or political. An example is the *UK Health For All Network*, whose members are committed to pursuing the WHO HFA 2000 strategy.[10]

In order to enter a particular network it may be necessary to identify the 'gatekeepers' who control entry, and other people who are influential in the network and could act as a sponsor for someone seeking to join. Having entered a network it is important to support the values and established ways of working. Later, having been accepted, it may be possible to challenge accepted practices.

Making Deals

Making deals is a common practice in most organisations. Individuals or groups agree to support a proposal in return for agreement on something which benefits them. In order to make deals successfully, it pays to know the person with whom you are dealing, paying careful attention to the values and intentions of the other party and what you could realistically expect from them.

On Being 'Political' . . .

A final point is about 'political' behaviour, by which we mean finding out about who holds power, and working to use this information to change a situation. When is it acceptable and when is it unethical?

Being 'political' can smack of being devious and manipulative. Many people view political behaviour with suspicion and will therefore not be easily influenced by it. Most people mistrust those who seek to manipulate covertly, or who coerce, lie, or deliberately withhold information which affects others. We do not support any of these tactics.

But to ignore the politics within organisations is unwise, because it results in failure to make a realistic appraisal of situations, and failure to make the best of the opportunities for positive health promotion. Furthermore, we contend that it is possible to be 'political' without losing professional integrity. For example, we suggest that deals are best made as the outcome of open negotiations, and that relationships should be based on genuineness, trust, goodwill and mutual respect.

Case Study: The politics of influence—health and safety at work

Bob is an environmental health officer working for Blackspot City Council. His aim is to improve the implementation of the health and safety at work policy of the council. He makes a list of the *helping* forces and the *hindering* forces:

Helping:

- the existing safety officers
- existing codes of practice, for example, sight checks for VDU operators
- a councillor who is a health lecturer at the Polytechnic
- a personnel officer interested in improving the working environment for staff
- an existing commitment to appoint an occupational health nurse

Hindering:

- the cost of any improvements (the council has severe financial constraints)
- staff time to attend health and safety training
- problems with recruiting an occupational health nurse
- deficiencies in the structure of council buildings (poor ventilation, open plan offices, lack of showers for those staff wishing to take physical exercise during the day)
- lack of councillors' commitment to improve health and safety conditions for staff
- lack of access to council buildings for disabled people

He identifies the stakeholders as:

- the staff themselves
- the trade unions
- departmental managers, senior and chief officers

continued on next page

continued

- the councillors
- the public health medicine department and the health promotion officer of the local district health authority

He further identifies key stakeholders as:

- officers in the department of engineering because they enforce building regulations
- council members on the health committee
- the director of personnel

He then identifies ways of increasing the helping forces and decreasing the hindering forces. Through making an ally of the interested personnel officer he is able to increase the commitment of the director of personnel, who is also a chief officer. One short-term outcome is that an occupational health nurse is recruited. Another outcome is a plan agreed by the personnel department and the trade unions for training staff in health and safety.

By joining a local network of people interested in health promotion he is able to find out what is going on elsewhere and this gives him some useful ideas, including sources of help in stress management training which he incorporates into the training plan.

He makes a deal with the engineering department by agreeing to assist with monitoring construction sites of new buildings in order to prevent accidents on the site. In return, they agree to assist with a plan for improving soundproofing and modifications to open plan offices. Their commitment grows after a report shows that accidents on construction sites are reduced. He discusses with them the issue of raising with council members the plan for modifying council buildings.

Finally, he makes an ally of the councillor at the Polytechnic by offering to provide an input to some of the courses. This councillor is on the health committee and provides him with useful advice on how to approach the committee and how to prepare documents for its consideration.

Developing and Implementing Policies

Many health promoters have a role in developing and implementing policies, often policies about health issues which relate to workplaces. For some health issues, policies are common practice, and there are practical guidelines and model policies available; policies on smoking at work are probably one of the best examples.[11] In other areas, such as policies on AIDS, work is less developed.[12]

Policies on Promoting Health in the Workplace

For general workplace policies, WHO has provided policy guidance.[13] WHO has adopted a broad concept of well-being in the workplace, which includes how work is organised, managerial styles and communication at work, working conditions, job design and type of work. It is clear that health promotion in the workplace could result in considerable improvements in health. Leading employers and trade unions have begun to take on a wider concept of health at work, including giving priority to issues such as smoking, alcohol and stress. WHO guidance is in line with the recommendations of a Health Education Authority report.[14] The recommendations of this report include:

- setting targets for the reduction of illness in the working population;
- changes in workplace policies, working practices and individual lifestyles to reduce the risk of ill-health and promote well-being of workers;
- systematic elimination of hazardous exposures and sources of unhealthy stress in the workplace.

The Health and Safety Executive is a source of information on all regulations governing health and safety in the workplace.[15]

Developing and Implementing Workplace Policies

The process of developing and implementing a health promotion workplace policy involves four stages—preparation, implementation, education and training, and evaluation.[16] We shall now consider each of these in turn.

Preparation of the policy. The formulation of a policy by any organisation is a corporate matter, so the usual starting point is to convene a working group. This group:

- clarifies its terms of reference and elects a chairperson;
- identifies the need for a policy;
- identifies the committee, department or senior officer who has overall responsibility for taking the policy forward;
- identifies key personnel to be consulted and convinced of the need for a policy;
- establishes a timescale for policy development;
- prepares a draft policy and consults widely;
- prepares the final draft policy for approval.

In the case of a workplace policy, it is important to involve the trade unions. This can be achieved either by including trade union representatives on the working group or by setting up an effective framework for consultation and negotiation. This may be crucial in persuading the workforce to look positively on the new policy.

It is also important that an identified senior officer or manager, with political 'clout', acts as a 'champion' for the policy. This person will be crucial in getting the commitment of other managers to the policy.

Implementing the policy. This begins with planning, which will include:

- setting aims and objectives
- setting up a system for monitoring and evaluation
- identifying resources and defining key implementation tasks

- defining the role of key personnel
- developing an action plan.

Key personnel should be encouraged to participate actively in identifying their roles and in discussing boundaries and overlap of roles so that the potential for conflict and confusion is reduced. For example, managers have primary responsibility for ensuring that their staff are fully conversant with workplace policies and understand what is expected of them. Nevertheless, the trade unions also have a role in informing the workforce of the policy. These sources of information will, one hopes, be complementary and spell out the same and not contradictory messages. Open discussion of these issues will help to increase commitment to making the policy work.

Any policy which is not the subject of regular review risks becoming obsolete. So the working group must reconvene at regular intervals to consider issues such as:

- does the workforce know about and understand the policy?
- have attitudes to the health issue covered by the policy changed and if so how? How do staff feel about the policy?
- has the behaviour of individual staff changed? Does this include changes in working practices and/or individual lifestyles?
- do staff get any help they may need?
- do managers and trade unions support the policy?
- do indicators show that the policy is making progress towards the attainment of its aims and objectives? For example, has absenteeism and sickness been reduced? Or have accident rates decreased? Has work performance improved? Is morale better?
- how can the effectiveness of the policy be improved?

Education and training. This is a continuous process not a one-off event. Wherever possible it should be integrated into existing provision for professional and managerial staff development. The purposes of education and training include:

- securing the commitment of management, for example, of elected members, chief officers and senior management in the case of a local authority;
- obtaining the commitment of the whole workforce;
- providing those responsible for implementing the policy with the necessary skills;
- overcoming prejudices, discrimination and stereotyping where relevant (for example in policies on alcohol and HIV/AIDS);
- encouraging and assisting the workforce in making choices and individual lifestyle changes.

Evaluation. This should include evaluation of both process and outcomes. It will require the collection of information, both base-line and on-going. See the section *Plan evaluation methods* in Chapter Six for further suggestions.

For information on policy formulation for specific target groups, health issues and situations, see the suggestions at the end of this chapter.[17]

Exercise—A workplace alcohol policy

Bloggshire Health Authority is participating in a regional programme on sensible drinking. As part of this programme, organisations such as health authorities within the region are encouraged to develop policies on alcohol for their workforce.

The District Health Promotion Officer for Bloggshire Health Authority therefore convenes a working group to develop a policy, which includes representatives of personnel officers, general management, consultant psychiatrists, trade unions and the local voluntary organisation on alcohol misuse.

The working group meets four times, and produces a draft policy. The policy specifies that the Authority sees sensible drinking as everyone's responsibility and that all employees will receive basic information about sensible drinking. It also covers the Authority's responsibility to develop an environment conductive to self-referral by anyone with an alcohol problem, early identification of alcohol-related problems and the provision of expert confidential help. It looks at the provision of alcohol on Authority premises, and specifies that non-alcoholic drink should be provided as an alternative at all social functions where alcohol is served, and that alcohol consumption should be discouraged at non-social functions.

This draft policy goes to the Health Authority's Health Promotion Committee. It receives a lukewarm reception, and there is much concern that it will interfere with personnel policies on dealing with people who drink on duty. There is also discussion and disagreement about what constitutes 'social' and 'non-social' functions, and resistance to the idea of curtailing 'social' drinking, ie. selling alcohol at the doctors' bar, and serving it at working lunches, publicity events such as the opening of new clinics, and leaving parties.

Nevertheless, it is passed for consultation, and comes back to the Committee for final approval. The Committee are still unenthusiastic, and one major change they make alters the working group's recommendations on implementation. These were that many departments and officers had a key role, including personnel, health promotion, general management and training departments. This is changed so that responsibility for implementation rests entirely with the District Personnel Officer. The Alcohol Policy is finally approved formally by the Health Authority.

Soon after this, the Health Promotion Committee (which had a remit to monitor health promotion policies) is abolished in a major health service reorganisation. There follows a long period of massive organisational change. Three years after the original working group met, the alcohol policy has never been implemented. There has been no education of the workforce about 'sensible drinking' and no change in the way alcohol is served and sold on health authority premises.

Looking at the stages for developing and implementing a workplace policy in the section above, and the section on 'The politics of influence', consider:

- what steps were taken which helped the policy development?
- what else could have been done?

continued on next page

continued

- why did the policy receive such a lukewarm reception by the Health Promotion Committee? Could anything have been done to prevent this?
- why was the policy never implemented? Could anything have been done to ensure that the implementation stage actually happened?
- are there any other significant points to note about the lessons learnt from this case study?

Campaigning

You, or clients with whom you work, may feel strongly about changing policy or practice about a health issue, and decide that the way forward is to mount a *campaign*.[18]

Campaigns can range from short-lived local ones with the objective of making a single change ('save our local cottage hospital') to long-term national ones such as 'Keep Britain Tidy' or annual 'drinking and driving' campaigns. *Pressure groups* are made up of the people who are running the campaign, such as the 'Save our Cottage Hospital Campaign Group'. Examples of national pressure groups are 'Shelter' (on homelessness) or 'Friends of the Earth' (on environmental issues). Some pressure groups (like 'Shelter') may also provide direct services as well as acting as a pressure group.

Principles of Campaigning

Some important principles to be kept in mind if you are setting up a campaign are:[19]

- **be persistent:** success requires persistent effort, so you must be committed and prepared to put in a lot of time and energy over as long a period as necessary—which may be a very long time.
- **be professional:** give care and attention to details (such as well-written letters, preferably typed, with the name of the campaign clearly evident) and ensure that activities such as keeping records are undertaken properly.
- **keep a sense of perspective:** your campaign may be vitally important to you, but being perceived as a fanatical crank (or even *being* a fanatical crank!) will do your cause no good.
- **reflect your ideas in your behaviour:** it is no good, for example, campaigning to clean up your neighbourhood if your own front garden looks like a tip. Nor is it helpful to campaign for equal opportunities if the place where your own organisation meets has no access for the disabled.
- **be positive:** for example, call yourselves the 'Save the Cottage Hospital Campaign Group' rather than 'Group Against Closing the Cottage Hospital'. For example, 'Shelter' is called the 'National Campaign *for* the Homeless', not the 'Campaign *against* Bad Housing'.
- **join with others:** rival pressure groups campaigning on similar (or even identical) issues waste a lot of time and effort. If someone is already campaigning on 'your' issue, join them rather than set up a rival organisation. Or, if there is more than one organisation working on similar issues, form a coalition. For example, the 'Save the

Cottage Hospital Campaign Group' could link with the local Community Health Council if its members are also concerned about the issue.

- **where you can, do something as you go along:** for example, if you are campaigning to clean up your neighbourhood, you could organise a one-off 'Litter Collection Day' as well as lobbying your local council for better refuse collection and more litter bins.
- **involve as many people as possible:** this is not only to harness their support but to enable people to see for themselves what is wrong and what needs to change.

Planning a Campaign

When you plan a campaign, it helps to go through the same planning process as you would with any other kind of health promotion activity (see also Chapter Six *Planning and Evaluating*):

- identify your aims clearly
- decide the best way of achieving them (eg. public meetings? press coverage? lobbying MPs and local councillors? getting up a petition?)
- identify your resources (do you need to fund-raise?)
- clarify how you will know if your aim is achieved (eg. when the local health authority promises to reconsider the closure of the hospital or when the authority has formally agreed to keep it open for a specified length of time?)
- set an action plan of who is going to what and when.

Implementing Change

People react very differently to change for a variety of reasons. While one person passively resists a change, another may actively try to sabotage it, whereas a third may actually get involved in bringing it about. Whether you are campaigning for a change, or implementing a change in policy or practice in your work, you will need to deal with the fact that many people resist change for a number of reasons, including:

- **Self interest**—while a change may be in the interest of most people, it may not be in *everyone's* best interest. For example, while most people, including some smokers, may support an anti-smoking policy, others may see it as an infringement of personal liberty and not in their interest.
- **Misunderstanding**—people can easily misunderstand what is being proposed. For example, people may misunderstand an alcohol policy and think that it is letting people with drinking problems 'off the hook', so that they do not have to meet the same standards of work performance and behaviour as everyone else. Misunderstandings are particularly frequent in organisations where there is a lack of trust between the managers and the workforce.
- **Belief that a change is not in the interest of the people it is intended to benefit**—people may believe that the costs of a change will outweigh the benefits, not only to themselves, but to other people or to a whole organisation. For example, people may feel that the introduction of ethnic monitoring as part of an equal

opportunities policy could actually increase discrimination against black and other minority ethnic groups. Awareness of these opinions is important for the policy-maker, because they may be based on knowledge of what goes on in parts of the organisation with which the policy maker has little contact. Policy information must be based on accurate analysis of the situation; this is particularly relevant in large organisations, like the Health Service and county councils.

- **Low tolerance for change**—people may resist change because they are anxious about new demands which will be made of them. For example, there may be demands to provide separate rest rooms for smokers, or health counselling for people with alcohol problems. Organisational change can require people to change too much, or fail to provide them with the time and support they need.

Methods for Overcoming Resistance to Change

In order to overcome resistance to change it is vital to select the best approach, or combination of approaches, for the situation and the people involved. Five possible options are:

1. **Education and communication**—this involves educating people about a change before it happens and communicating with them in a variety of ways—one-to-one, group discussion, written documents, etc. An educational and communication approach is indicated when resistance to change is based on inadequate or inaccurate information. The limitation is that it can be time-consuming, especially if many people are involved.
2. **Participation and involvement**—resistance to change may be forestalled if those initiating the change identify the people who they think will be resistant, and actively involve them in the process of designing and implementing the change. The initiators of the change must genuinely be prepared to listen and learn. A token effort is liable to provoke more resistance, because people will feel tricked if their advice is not heeded. Participation and involvement is indicated when people need to be committed to a policy change in order to make it work; policies work when people feel a sense of ownership of them because they have been involved in their development. This approach is also useful when the initiators do not have full information about the implications of the change for certain groups of people or certain departments. It could also be the preferred option where the initiators of change have little power, because it harnesses the power of others as a force for change. Nevertheless, this approach does have limitations. It is very time-consuming and demands a high degree of co-ordination, and it can lead to a poor outcome if it tries to please everybody.
3. **Facilitation and support**—this involves helping people to identify what changes are required and providing them with support to plan and manage the change themselves. This can be done, for example, by providing 'time out' for people to reflect on the situation, and to identify their own objectives and how to meet them. Support can include emotional support to cope with stress and 'burn out', and the development of 'mentoring' or 'facilitator' schemes, where more experienced people help others with their managerial or professional development. This approach works best where anxiety and fear lie at the heart of resistance. The limitation of this

approach is that it, too, can be time-consuming and expensive (for example, if it is necessary to employ counsellors for a large workforce).

4. **Negotiation and agreement**—this involves offering incentives to actual or potential resisters, for example, through negotiating with trade unions about the effects of the change on their members' pay. This is particularly appropriate when it is obvious that some people will lose out as a consequence of the changes. It can be effective if there are specific pockets of resistance, but could be expensive if everyone leaps on the bandwagon and tries to argue that they are also losing out.
5. **Political influencing**—this approach has already been discussed. It can be useful where one, or a few, very powerful individuals are the source of resistance. It can be relatively quick, but has the drawback that it can lead to problems in the future if people feel that they have been manipulated.

Notes, References and Further Reading

1 For example, in Devon the Local Education Authority and the Exeter Health Authority have agreed to jointly fund a secondary school adviser for health education. This has helped with the co-ordination of health education across the school curriculum.

See also:

Simnett I (1991) *Promoting Health—Local Authorities in Action.* London: Health Education Authority

2 DHSS (1989) *United Kingdom's Monitoring Report on the Strategy for Health For All by the Year 2000* (1985–1988). London: DHSS

3 See, for example:

National Children's Bureau (1987) A Report of the Policy and Practice Review Group *Investing in the Future—Child Health Ten Years after the Court Report.* London: National Children's Bureau

The Health Promotion Authority for Wales has been carrying out regular surveys of school health policy, including how health education is organised, what policies there are in the school environment, and the extent of family and school links. See:

Nutbeam D *et al* (1987) The Health Promoting School: organisation and policy development in Welsh secondary schools. *Health Education Journal*, **46**, 109–115

The Health Education Authority collaborates with a variety of bodies in the area of policy development. See, for example:

Health Education Authority, Alcohol Concern and the National Health Service Training Authority (1988) *Guidelines for Health Authorities on the Development, Implementation and Evaluation of an Alcohol Policy for their Staff.* Available from the HEA

4 Secretary of State for Health (1991) *The Health of the Nation: a Consultative Document for Health in England.* London: HMSO

5 For case studies of politics and power in health promotion, see:

Rodmell S & Watt A (eds) (1986) *The Politics of Health Education—Raising the Issues*. London: Routledge & Kegan Paul

Cannon G (1987) *The Politics of Food*. London: Century

Jacobson B (1988) *Beating the Ladykillers*. London: Gollancz (On the politics of tobacco with reference to women smoking.)

6 You can find out who your MP and local councillor are, and details of their 'surgeries', from libraries and Citizens Advice Bureaux. You can write to your MP at:

The House of Commons, Westminster, London SW1A 0AA (Telephone: 071 219 3000)

7 For an introduction to power and influence see:

Handy C B (1985) *Understanding Organisations*. Harmondsworth: Penguin Business Books, Ch 5

For a comprehensive theory of power and the relationship between power, influence and authority, see:

Mintzberg H (1983) *Power In and Around Organisations*. London: Prentice-Hall

8 This section is partly based on:

Kakabadse A P (1982) The politics of interpersonal influence. In *Leadership and Organisation Development* 3, No. 3. Bradford: MCB University Press

9 Darling J R (1985) Managing up in the multi-national firm. *Leadership and Organisational Development Journal*, 7, 1

For more on influencing people, see:

Bolton R & Bolton D G (1984) *Social Style/Management Style*. New York: American Management Association

10 For further information on the UK Health For All Network, contact:

UK Health For All Network, PO Box 101, Liverpool L69 5BE. Telephone: 051 231 1009.

Other health promotion networks include:

The Public Health Alliance, PO Box 1156, Kings Norton, Birmingham B30 2AZ

The Local Authorities Health Network, PO Box 103, Chesterfield, Derbyshire S44 5UB. Telephone: 0246 851143

11 See:

Jenkins M *et al.* (1987) *Smoking Policies at Work*. London: Health Education Authority

Health Education Council (1985) *Action on Smoking at Work: a Guide to Good Practice*. London: Health Education Council

Batten L (1990) *Managing Change: Smoking Policies in the NHS*. London: Health Education Authority

12 Beardshaw V, Hunter D J & Taylor R C R (1990) *Local AIDS Policies: Planning and Policy Development for Health Promotion* AIDS Programme Papers No. 6. London: Health Education Authority

13 World Health Organisation (1988) *Health Promotion for Working Populations*. Report of a WHO Expert Committee; Technical Report Series No. 765. Geneva: WHO

14 Webb A *et al* (1988) *Health at Work? A Report on Health Promotion in the Workplace*. Research Report No. 22. London: Health Education Authority

15 Health and Safety Executive, Baynards House, 1 Chepstow Place, Westbourne Grove, London W2 4TF. Telephone: 071 221 0870

16 This is based on:

Simnett I & Chiles M (1989) *A Practical Guide to Developing and Implementing Alcohol Policies*. Frenchay Health Authority and:

Health and Consumer Service, Sheffield City Council (1989) *Guidelines for Local Authorities on the Development, Implementation and Evaluation of an Alcohol Policy for their Staff*. London: Health Education Authority

17 For further information on policy related to child health, see:

Faculty of Community Medicine (1987) *An Integrated Child Health Service: the Way Forward*. London: Faculty of Community Medicine

For further information on policy related to sexuality, see:

Allen I (1987) *Education in Sex and Personal Relationships*. London: Policy Studies Institute

Massey D (1988) *School Sex Education: Why, What and How?* London: Family Planning Association

For policy development related to the development of burn and scald accidents in children, see:

Child Accident Prevention Trust (1985) *Burn and Scald Accidents to Children*. London: Bedford Square Press

For further information on developing school policies, see:

Scottish Health Education Group/Scottish Consultative Council on the Curriculum (1989) *Promoting Good Health*. Edinburgh: SHEG/SCCC

Reid D J (1985) The prevention of smoking among schoolchildren: recommendations for policy development. *Health Education Journal*, **44**, 3–12

For further information on policies for older people, see:

Norton A *et al* (1986) *Councils of Care: Planning a Local Government Strategy for Older People*. Policy Studies in Ageing No. 5. London: Centre for Policy on Ageing

For information on policy development related to educational opportunities for the elderly, see:

Open University/UDACE (1988) *Learning Later*. Available from: Community Education Development Centre, Lyng Hall, Blackberry Lane, Coventry CV2 3JS

For further information on local food health policies in the UK, see

Gibson L & Champion P (1989) *Survey of Local Food Health Policies in the UK*. Department of Social Policy, Cranfield Institute of Technology/ NHSTA/HEA. London: Health Education Authority

For further information on policies related to the prevention of cervical cancer, see:

Parkin D M & Moss S M (1986) An evaluation of screening policies for cervical cancer in England and Wales using a computer-simulated model. *Journal of Epidemiology & Community Health*, **40**, 143–153

For further information on health promotion policies of Regional Health Authorities, see:

Castle P & Jacobson B (1988)*The Health of our Regions: an Analysis of the Strategies and Policies of Regional Health Authorities for Promoting Health and Preventing Disease*. A Report for the Health Education Authority. Birmingham: NHS Regions Health Promotion Group

Also see notes 9, 10 and 11 above.

18 For a practical guide to campaigning, see:

Bird P (1989) *How To Run a Local Campaign: a Step-by-step Manual for Organisers*. London: Northcote House Publishers

19 This section is adapted from some material in Chapter 2 of:

Wilson D (1984) *Pressure: the A to Z of Campaigning in Britain*. London: Heinemann. The whole of this book is recommended for further reading.

See also:

Davies M (1985) *Politics of Pressure*. London: British Broadcasting Corporation

Chapter 14
Using and Producing Health Promotion Materials

Summary

Some principles governing the choice of health promotion materials are suggested in the first part of the chapter. This is followed by a summary of the uses, advantages and limitations of the main types of teaching and learning materials. The last section in the chapter outlines points for making the most of display materials, for producing written materials (including guidance on non-sexist writing), and for presenting statistical information. The chapter includes exercises on the 'Gobbledygook Test', writing plain English and presenting statistics in visual ways.

Teaching materials and learning aids such as leaflets, posters and videos are used extensively in the practice of health promotion.[1] But are they always used *effectively*? In this chapter we aim to give you information and guidelines to help you to choose, produce and use materials with maximum effectiveness.

Material resources are *adjuncts* to education, advice-giving, group work, community-based work or counselling. *How* resources are used is as crucial as the quality of the resources themselves.

Health Promotion Materials: Criteria for Choice

There is a huge range of materials available, with a constant turnover as items become out of date or out of print and new ones come on the market. So you may find yourself with the task of selecting a leaflet, poster, display or video from a range of possibilities. Or you may find that there is very little available, and you have to decide whether the one item you have found is suitable.

The following guidelines are designed to help you to select the most appropriate and useful materials for displays, group teaching or for use with individual clients. The guidelines apply to selecting any kind of material, such as leaflets, posters or videos, and can also be used when you are producing your own materials.

Guidelines for Selecting and Producing Health Promotion Material

Is it appropriate for achieving your promotion aims? Think about the item in the context of how you intend to use it: for example, if you are working with a group of young smokers who are not motivated to stop, a leaflet or video on 'How to Stop Smoking' is unlikely to be helpful at this stage; materials to trigger discussion with the aim of challenging attitudes might be better. (See the section *Stage 3: Decide the best way of achieving the aims* in Chapter Six.)

Is it the most appropriate kind of material? Will another medium be better because it is more flexible (eg. will slides be better than a video because they can be edited)? Will something else be cheaper and just as effective (eg. photographs instead of a video?) Could the real thing be used instead of being portrayed via a teaching aid (eg. parents in person talking about their experiences of a new baby instead of appearing in a video, babies instead of dolls, actual foods instead of pictures or models?).

Is it consistent with your values and approach? If your approach is to work in a non-judgmental partnership with your clients, the materials you use should reflect your values. So you need to avoid material which is patronising, authoritarian or scaremongering, for example. (See the section *Exploring relationships with clients* in Chapter Eight.)

Material should not be 'victim blaming'. That is, it should not attribute blame to individuals who are ill when their ill-health is rooted in their social circumstances, for example, poverty or bad housing.

Is it relevant for the people you are working with? Does the material reflect the values and culture of your clients? Does it reflect their concerns? Does it take into account their age, ethnic group, sex and socioeconomic status? Does it reflect local practice and conditions and the health services available? Obvious examples of irrelevance are videos portraying American lifestyles, or the homes of affluent middle-class families, which may both be irrelevant if you are working with people in the UK who are not well-off. Another example is that of materials designed for one ethnic group that may not be appropriate for another, not just because of language but because some aspects (such as sexual behaviour or attitudes to bereavement) may be seen very differently in different cultures.

Is it racist or sexist? All material should be non-racist. Racist material is that which stereotypes people into racial types, attributing certain roles or character attributes on the basis of ethnic group alone. Implicit in this are the assumptions that one ethnic group (usually white, Caucasian or European) is superior to another, and one ethnic group (usually white), represents the desired 'norm'. (For some useful references on racism, see note 3 at the end of Chapter Eight.)

All material should be non-sexist. Sexist material is that which stereotypes men and women into certain roles or character attributes on the basis of gender. In particular, it is any portrayal of women as sex objects for the gratification of men, any trivialisation or demeaning of women as second-class citizens, dependent on their relationships with men for social status, and any assumption that male equals desirable norm, whereas female equals undesirable deviant. (We provide guidance on non-sexist writing later in this chapter.)

Material should reflect the fact that we live in a multiracial society where the roles of men and women are changing. Strong, positive messages and images should be provided of people of all ethnic groups and both sexes.

Will it be understood? Is the material in plain English which people will readily understand? (There is more about writing plain English and assessing readability later in this chapter.) Are there any incorrect assumptions about the level of literacy or existing knowledge? Does it need to be produced in other languages, to make it accessible to people from minority ethnic groups?

Is the information sound? Is information in the materials accurate, up-to-date, unbiased and complete? Or does it contain half-truths, one-sided information on controversial issues, and out-of-date or incomplete messages?

Does it contain advertising? Much material is produced by commercial companies such as drug companies, non-NHS companies offering health and fitness checks, baby food manufacturers or makers of safety equipment. Material (leaflets and posters, for example) usually carries the name of the company or its products, or includes advertisements. Using these materials can imply that you (or your employing agency) are endorsing the product. It may also damage your image as a credible source of unbiased health information, and lead people to doubt the value of the information ('they're just trying to sell me something').

For these reasons, material containing company names, products and advertising should be avoided whenever possible. However, it may be just what you want, and there may be no alternative. In this case, we suggest that:

- the product or service advertised must be ethically acceptable as 'healthy' and 'environmentally friendly'. This excludes tobacco, alcohol and confectionery advertising, for example;
- the advertising content must be low-key. The company name on the front or back cover is acceptable, but constant references to named brand products are not.

The Range of Materials—Uses, Advantages and Limitations

There is a wide range of materials available to you, some of which may be more familiar than others. We would like to emphasise two points by way of introduction; the first is that teaching aids are *aids* and not substitutes for the teacher. Videos, for example, are easily misused by being presented without an introduction or with no follow-up discussion and shown just because 'it is a good video'. Secondly, it takes time and practice to become familiar and comfortable with all the aids available, and it takes courage to try out new things—but it is worth it.

The following summary briefly outlines the uses, advantages and limitations of the main types of aid. Further reading for more detailed information is given at the end of this chapter, but reading is no substitute for practice and experiment.[2]

Leaflets, Handouts and Other Written Materials

Uses and Advantages

1 Allow client self-pacing and self-teaching.
2 Consumers can 'revise' the content of health teaching at their leisure.
3 Information can be shared with relatives and friends.
4 Can give further details (eg. statistics) which would clutter up a talk.
5 Handouts are easily produced, duplicated and revised, and therefore easily updated.
6 Handouts can reduce the need for note-taking.
7 Handouts and non-commercially produced leaflets can be cheap.
8 Clients and educator can work through complex information together.

Limitations

1 Professionally-produced leaflets can be expensive.
2 Mass-produced material is designed for the average consumer, and is not always suitable for everybody.
3 Commercially-produced material may contain advertising.
4 Leaflets and handouts are not durable and are easily lost.
5 Handouts demand good typing and reproducing facilities.
6 Pre-testing with the consumer group is advisable.
7 Can end up as unread waste paper unless the educator actively involves the client in reading and using the material.

Posters and Charts

Uses and Advantages

1 Can raise awareness of health issues, and challenge beliefs, attitudes and behaviour.
2 Can convey information, direct people to other sources (addresses, telephone numbers, 'pick up a leaflet').
3 Can be 'home-made' cheaply.

Limitations

1 For small audiences only (except giant commercial posters).
2 Quickly get damaged, tatty and ignored.
3 High-quality material needs trained graphic artists and good printing equipment. This can be expensive.
4 Can be relatively expensive to buy.
5 Pre-testing with the consumer group advisable.

Videotapes

Uses and Advantages

1 Convey reality (movement, sound, places, emotion) which may otherwise be inaccessible to the audience (eg. childbirth).
2 Can convey information, pose problems, demonstrate skills.
3 Can trigger discussion on attitudes and behaviour.
4 Suitable for medium and small audiences.
5 Can be used for self-teaching and will permit self-pacing.
6 Can easily be stopped and started to permit discussion between sections. Sections can be replayed for detailed analysis.
7 Educational programmes for TV can be recorded for later use.
8 Packages including discussion notes and worksheets are produced to link with educational TV programmes.
9 Video equipment is becoming increasingly cheap and available.
10 Little or no blackout required.
11 Equipment relatively simple to use.

Limitations

1 Electricity supply and costly equipment required.
2 Equipment can break down.
3 There are problems with the compatibility of different types of videos and equipment.
4 Copyright regulations for videotaping TV programmes are not always clear and may be restrictive.
5 Small size of screen limits size of audience.

Slides

Uses and Advantages

1 Go some way towards conveying reality.
2 Can convey information, pose problems, demonstrate skills.
3 Can trigger discussion on attitudes and behaviour.
4 Suitable for all sizes of audience including very large ones.
5 Relatively cheap and easy to produce.
6 Cheap to buy.
7 Sets of slides can be edited to suit particular audiences.
8 Can be used for self-teaching, which permits self-pacing.
9 Equipment light and easy to transport.
10 Equipment easy to use.

Limitations

1 Electricity and fairly costly equipment required.

2 Equipment can break down (but comparatively little to go wrong).
3 Needs at least partial darkness for viewing (unless special daylight screen available).

Audiotapes

Uses and Advantages

1 Especially suited to self-teaching and small groups.
2 Can be stopped and started easily to facilitate discussion.
3 Can convey information, pose problems, trigger discussion.
4 Good for certain skills development, eg. relaxation, exercise routines.
5 Cheap.
6 Equipment widely available.
7 Can be linked to slides to make tape/slide sets—much cheaper and easier to make than videos.

Limitations

1 Good quality recording requires studio facilities.
2 Do not hold attention as well as visual material.
3 There can be problems with acoustics.

Overhead Projector Transparencies

Uses and Advantages

1 Can be used to build up information by overlaying one or more transparencies.
2 Can be prepared in advance or used to note points while teaching.
3 Educator faces audience and maintains rapport.
4 Can be used with any size of audience.
5 Cheap to buy.
6 Cheap and easy to home-produce.
7 No blackout needed.
8 Equipment relatively cheap.
9 Equipment easy to use and maintain.
10 Equipment widely available and portable overhead projectors are available.

Limitations

1 Difficult to introduce movement into visuals.
2 Ideally should have a sloping screen—otherwise the projected image is wider at the top than the bottom, and is not equally focused.
3 The lens assembly of the overhead projector can obstruct the view of the screen from some positions—careful seating arrangements are therefore necessary.
4 Requires an electricity supply.
5 Overhead projector can break down—eg. the bulb can blow.

Blackboards and Whiteboards (Wet-wipe and Dry-wipe)

Uses and Advantages

1 Good for structuring a topic and building up information in stages.
2 Good for highlighting/explaining particular points.
3 Nothing to break down!
4 No blackout needed.
5 Cheap and easily available.
6 Easily cleaned and re-used.
7 Whiteboards are easier to clean than blackboards and provide a better background for colour.
8 Permanent outlines can be drawn on whiteboards.

Limitations

1 Too small for groups of more than 25.
2 The educator has to turn her back on the audience when she writes on the board —may lose rapport.
3 Dry-wipe boards are easy to damage through incorrect cleaning—this results in shadow marking.

Flip-charts

Uses and Advantages

1 Good for brainstorming and for active involvement of a group in producing ideas which can be stuck up round the room for discussion.
2 Pages can be prepared in advance or used during teaching for notes and diagrams.
3 Easily portable—can be rolled or folded.
4 Can be used in rooms where there is no blackboard or whiteboard.
5 Cheap.
6 Nothing to break down.
7 No blackout needed.

Limitations

1 Too small for groups of more than 25.
2 Easily get torn and dog-eared.
3 Educator has to turn her back on the audience to write—may lose rapport.

Producing Materials

Most materials, particularly posters, leaflets and audiovisual materials, come ready-made, but you may want to work with a community group to help them to produce their own materials, or produce some yourself. We have not attempted to give a comprehensive guide on how to produce materials, but approaching the task in a systematic way using the *Planning and evaluation flowchart* in Chapter Six may be helpful. If you are producing a leaflet or poster, for example, you will need to consider who will write the draft, who will edit it, whether and how to pilot the draft, what it will cost and whether you need the services of a designer, illustrator, translater, typesetter or printer.

We have identified some important points for making the most effective posters, displays and written materials, as follows:

Making the Most of Display Materials

Posters, charts, display boards and stands.[3]

Be brief and to the point, keeping the objective firmly in mind. Do not include material which is irrelevant—it will only serve to distract from the main message.

Emphasise the key point(s) by altering the size of lettering, the style or colour. Place them just above the centre of a display, which is the point of maximum visual impact.

Use language the audience understands; explain any unfamiliar technical terms. If possible, express the message in both pictures and words. Test it out on a few people to ensure that you have no unexpected ambiguities in your message (eg. does the phrase 'beating heart disease' refer to information about how to avoid getting heart disease, or is it information on a health problem known as beating-heart disease?)

Be bold. Words and pictures should be as large as possible.

Make the most of colour. It can create continuity; for example, a repetition of background colour can link a series of posters. Colour can be used to identify parts of a diagram or highlight important information. Choose colours with care, because responses to colour are emotional, eg. blue is cool, green is soothing, and because colours may be associated with certain messages, images and places, eg. red for danger, purple for funerals, white for clinical cleanliness.

Improve the display site. If all you have is a blank wall or a wall covered with a distractingly-patterned wallpaper, fix a rectangle of coloured card to the wall as a background display board. If a display board has a rough or marked surface, give it a coat of paint or a covering of coloured paper, hessian or felt.

Use the display site to best advantage. Busy corridors can only be useful sites for posters with immediate appeal and few words. More information can be conveyed in a waiting area and it may be possible to supplement displays with leaflets to take away. Ensure that writing on displays is at eye level and large enough to be read without having to move from the queue or the chair.

Be aware of lighting. Daylight is unreliable, and spotlights directed on to a display are ideal.

Making Written Materials

Instruction sheets and cards, leaflets and booklets.[4]

Always test materials on a sample of consumers. Do not *assume* that you know what they like, want or need—*ask them.*

Note the use of colour, layout and print size to improve clarity. Large print may be helpful for the elderly.

Use plain English, simple words and short sentences. Use the active tense rather than the passive tense, eg. say 'change the bandage . . .' rather than 'the bandage should be changed . . .'

Do a Gobbledygook readability test on your written materials.[5] The test is a rough measure of readability for adult readers based on the principle that, by and large, the combination of long sentences and polysyllabic words is harder to comprehend. It is nonetheless also important to note that many other factors which affect readability, such as sentence structure, print size and the educational background of the reader, are not taken into account.

The Gobbledygook Test

This test is based on R. Gunning's FOG (Frequency of Gobbledygook) formula and was adapted by the Plain English Campaign.

This is what you do:

- Count a 100 word sample.
- Count the number of complete sentences in the sample.
- Count the total number of words in the complete sentences.
- Divide the number of words by the number of sentences. This gives the average sentence length.
- Count the number of words with three or more syllables in the 100 words. This gives the percentage of long words in the sample.
  Numbers and symbols are counted as short words; hyphenated words are counted as two words; a syllable, for the purposes of the test, is a vowel sound. So 'advised' is two syllables; 'applying' is three.
- Add the average sentence length to the percentage of long words to give the test score: the higher the score, the lower the 'readability'.

It is usual to do this three times to three different samples, one from the beginning of the text, one from the middle and one from near the end. These scores can then be added and divided by three to give the averge score.

continued on next page

continued

Tests carried out in 1980 by the National Consumer Council showed that the following publications had these scores:

Woman magazine	25
The Sun	26
Daily Mail	31
The Times	36
The Guardian	39

Exercise—The Gobbledygook Test

Do the Gobbledygook test on the following 100-word samples.

Sample 1

From now on, measures of alcohol will be stated in terms of beer, remembering that the alcohol content of all the following measures is roughly the same, so that statements made about, say, three pints of beer are also true of three doubles of spirit, or six glasses of wine, six glasses of sherry or two pints of special lager (which happens to be half as strong again as ordinary beer).

One has to consider, when trying to link intake of alcohol to the effects it has on individuals, that it is not only the amount of drink involved, but the . . .

Sample 2

We know that whooping cough vaccine works. The fact that there was so little whooping cough around when most children were immunised is one sign of how effective the vaccine is.

Remember that there are many different causes of brain damage in young children—many very much more common than whooping cough vaccine. In fact, the part played by whooping cough vaccine in causing any sort of brain damage at all is very tiny indeed.

Remember, too, that when doctors talk about brain damage, they do not necessarily mean severe mental handicap but usually something much less serious from which . . .

Exercise—Writing plain English

Write 'plain English' versions of the following. The first three are very similar to the instructions found on the packages of medication bought over the counter in chemist shops. The last three are very similar to passages in health education leaflets.

1. WHEEZOFF paediatric syrup is specially formulated for children. It is indicated for the relief of cough and its congestive symptoms and for the treatment of hay fever and other allergic conditions affecting the upper respiratory tract. Contraindications, warnings, etc.

continued on next page

continued

Hypersensitivity to any of the active constituents. If symptoms persist consult your doctor.

2. NOTWINGE cream—directions for use.
Apply a sufficient quantity of balm to the part affected. Massage lightly until penetration is complete.
3. SOOTHE vapour rub—how to apply.
Rub on chest, throat and back. Then spread it thick on chest. Repeat at bedtime. Leave bedclothes loose around the neck so that the decongestant antiseptic vapours may be inhaled freely. For severe nasal catarrh, head colds, coughs and bronchitis, melt some SOOTHE in boiling water and inhale the intensified decongestant antiseptic vapours.
4. If the room has a solid fuel, oil or gas-burning appliance ensure adequate ventilation.
5. The baby lies curled up in what is called the fetal position. It lies in a bag of water and the membranes which make up this fluid-filled balloon are enclosed in the womb.
6. Vitamin B1, also called thiamin, is required for the functioning of the nervous system, digestion and metabolism. Insufficient vitamin B1 can cause anorexia and fatigue.

Non-Sexist Writing[6]

We have already discussed the importance of material being non-racist and non-sexist, but using language in a non-sexist way presents particular challenges. One is the use of 'man' as a generic term for 'human beings'. For example, people talk about 'the working man' when workers are just as likely to be women. And 'manpower resources' are assumed to include both men and women, with the hidden assumption that women are second class resources. Many job titles end with 'man' and date from the time when only men performed these duties, for example, postman, ambulanceman. So it is important that, today, we choose words which reflect the reality of our situation. For example, instead of 'housewife' we can say 'houseworker'. The list below provides some more suggestions:

Change from:	*to:*
foreman	supervisor
salesman	sales associate, salesperson
repairman	repairer
manpower	workforce, staff, personnel
manning	staffing
ambulancemen	ambulance staff
newsman	newscaster, reporter

When *man* comes in the middle of a word, finding a one-word alternative can be difficult. Fortunately synonyms can usually be found; for example, instead of 'the carpenters did a workmanlike job', say 'the carpenters did a skilful job'.

Another problem is the generic use of the pronoun 'he'. For example 'Each doctor presented a case from his own practice', assumes that all the doctors are men. While it may seem clumsy to say 'he or she', it can sometimes usefully emphasise that both sexes are involved. An alternative is to turn the singular into a plural and use the words 'they' or 'their': 'The doctors presented cases from their own practices'. Similarly, instead of: 'A health promoter must be a fluent communicator. He must also be a good listener', say: 'Health promoters must be fluent communicators. They must also be good listeners'.

It may be possible to rephrase a passage to eliminate the pronouns altogether. So, instead of 'Information given to a social work agency is confidential in the same way as communications between a doctor and his patients', say '. . . in the same way as communications between doctors and patients'.

Another way is to use 'you' instead of 'he' or 'she' or a noun which implies male or female. For example, in a leaflet on parenting, you could change 'A mother often has difficulty in persuading her two-year-old to eat' to 'You may find it difficult to persuade your two-year-old to eat' or 'Parents may have difficulty . . .' This avoids the implication that it is only mothers (not fathers) who have a parenting role.

The use of 'he' can also be avoided by finding another noun. Thus, in 'You may find it difficult to persuade your two-year-old to eat. He may prefer throwing his food around instead' you could say '. . . A child at this age may prefer throwing food around instead'.

Sometimes, though, it seems impossible to avoid saying 'he' because the alternatives are clumsy or unclear. When we have found that to be the case in this book, we have chosen to use 'she' to denote a health promoter rather than 'he'. Many writers do this, thus challenging the tradition of using 'he' when meaning 'he or she'.

It is also important to avoid sexism when speaking as well writing. So, for instance, a consultant who refers to the women who attend for breast cancer screening (mammography) as 'the ladies' and the female radiographers as 'the girls' may intend no insult but it could offend both groups. It is far better to refer to the radiographers as 'the staff' ('girls' are women who have not yet grown up) and to the women who attend as 'women', 'patients' or 'clients'. You can test this by thinking how it would seem if you used the male equivalents (would you refer to men attending a clinic for testicular cancer as 'the gentlemen' and the staff attending them as 'the boys'?). (For further discussion of language barriers, see the section on this subject in Chapter Eight.)

Presenting Statistical Information

Numbers are useful for answering questions which begin how much? how many? how long? what's the risk? But numbers can be indigestible and meaningless unless they are carefully presented in a visual way.[7] The increasing availability of desk-top publishing and computer graphics means that it is becoming easier to produce information in ways which are visually arresting and easy to understand. Health and local authorities are likely to have the equipment and expertise to do this quite easily.

The following examples of a bar chart, pictogram, histogram and pie chart show how graphics can be used to bring a pictoral dimension to dry statistics.

The *Bar Chart* in Figure 10 shows how (1) people in different parts of the world and (2) men and women have different death rates from heart disease.

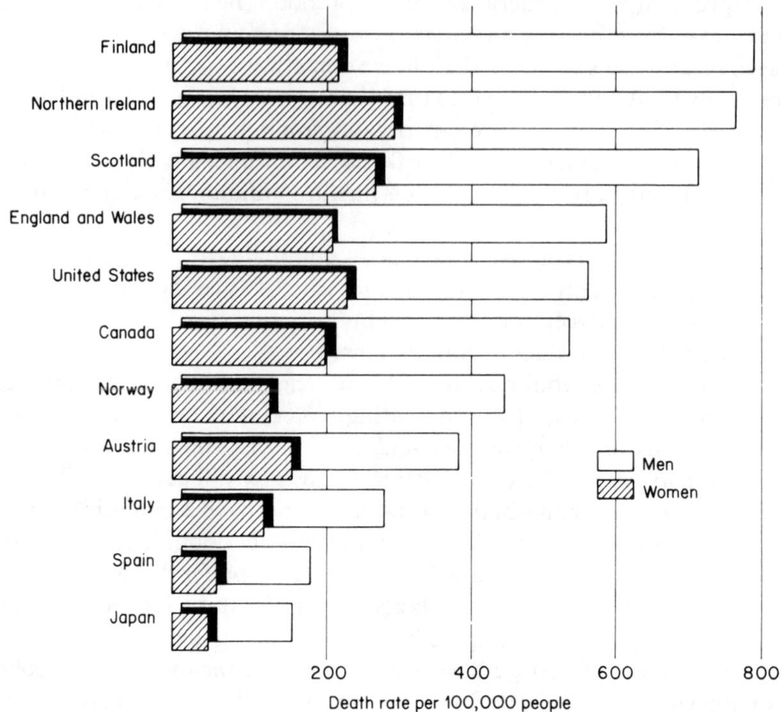

Fig. 10 Death rates from coronary heart disease in different countries (35–74 year olds). (Based on figures from the World Health Organisation.)[8]

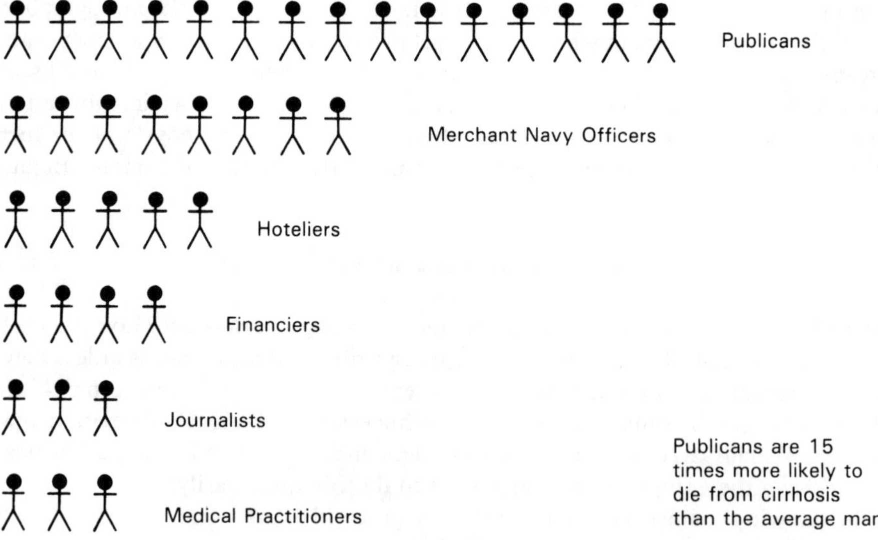

Fig. 11 Death rates (standardised mortality rates) from liver cirrhosis for selected occupations.[9]

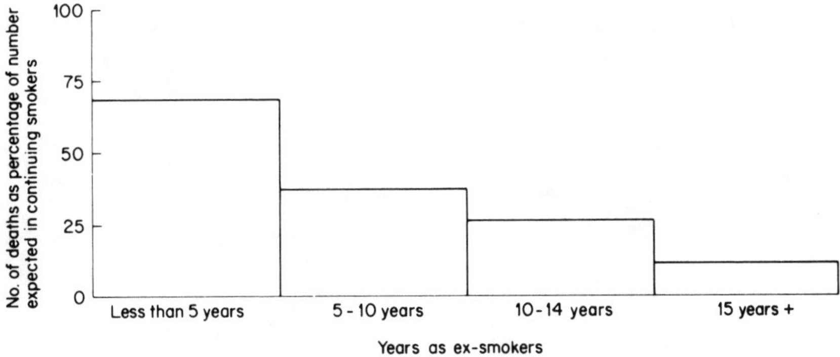

Fig. 12 The relationship between the number of years as an ex-smoker and death from lung cancer (in males).[10]

The *Pictogram* (Figure 11) shows how people in different occupations have different death rates from cirrhosis of the liver. A pictogram is similar to a bar chart but uses symbols to give greater visual effect.

The *Histogram* (Figure 12) shows how the ex-smoker's risk of dying from lung cancer gradually reduces with the passage of time. A histogram is a type of graph, which uses blocks rather than a curving line to simplify the presentation of the information.

The *Pie Chart* (Figure 13) shows the proportion of adults who smoke in England and Wales. A pie chart is a circle that is divided into segments (slices of the pie) so that the size of each segment is proportional to the number it represents. This example was calculated as follows:

Population of England and Wales = 41 million aged over 16 years
Number of smokers over 16 years = 15 million
41 million is represented by 360 degrees (ie. a full circle)
15 million is therefore represented by $\frac{360}{1} \times \frac{15}{41} = 131$ degrees

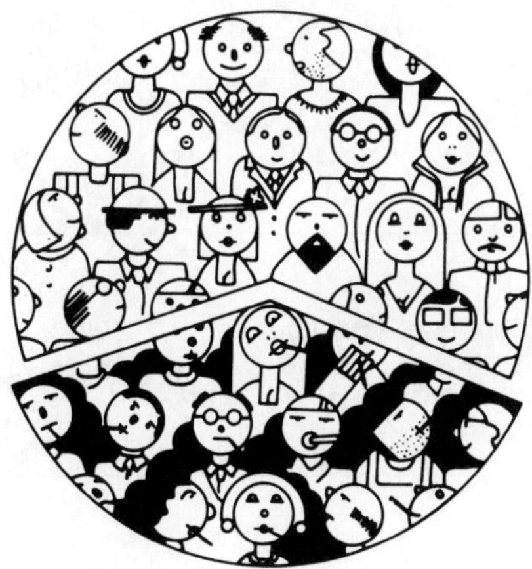

Fig. 13 The proportion of adults who smoke in England and Wales.[11]

Another *Pie Chart* (Fig. 14) illustrates that by far the greatest number of fatalities in drink-drive accidents are car occupants. The next biggest group are motorcyclists.

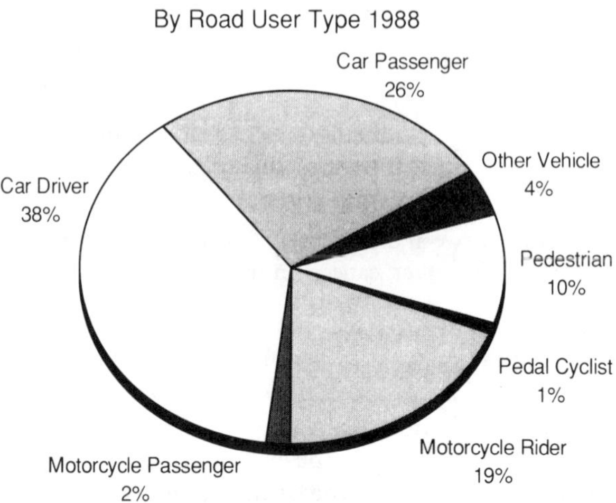

Fig. 14 Fatalities in drink-drive accidents.[12]

Exercise—Presenting statistical information

The following table gives statistics on the annual fatality rate from home accidents per 100,000 population in Great Britain.[13]

Age	Both sexes	Male	Female
0–14	3.5	3.9	3.1
15–64	5.2	6.0	4.2
65–74	19.6	19.0	19.7
74+	106.5	88.0	115.2

What key points of information can you identify?
Draw some sketches to show how you could present this information in a visual way.

Notes, References and Further Reading

1 Useful lists of health promotion resources are:

Health Education Authority resource lists covering a range of topics eg. food hygiene, mental health, smoking, HIV/AIDS; these are regularly updated. HEA, Hamilton House, Mabledon Place, London WC1H 9TX. Telephone: 071 383 3833

National Community Health Resource (NCHR) 15 Britannia Street, London WC1X 9JP. Telephone: 071 837 2426. This organisation provides support for community health initiatives, including books and teaching materials.

Health Education Index, published by Edsall, 124 Belgrave Road, London SW1V 2BL. This provides a comprehensive listing of health education materials. It is regularly updated.

2 Further reading on teaching aids:

Ellington H (1985) *Producing Teaching Materials*. London: Kogan Page. This includes chapters on displays, overhead projector transparencies, audio and videotapes and computer-mediated learning.

For a guide to producing and using leaflets effectively, see:

Pyle J & Harrington S (1988) *Making Leaflets Work: the Librarian's Guide to Effective Publicity*. The Publicity and Public Relations Group of the Library Association. Available from: Publicity and Publications Office, Central Library, Surrey Street, Sheffield S1 1XZ

For an introduction to video production for the non-specialist, see:

Fawbert F (no date) *Video Handbook*. Cambridge: National Extension College in association with the HEA and NHSTA. Available from: National Extension College, 18 Brooklands Avenue, Cambridge CB2 2HN. Telephone: 0223 3166443

3 For a guide to making displays interesting and effective, see:

McCann R (1988) *Graphics Handbook*. London: Health Education Authority/ National Extension College.

For a guide to desktop publishing (computerised integration of text and graphics), see:

Cookman B (1990) *Desktop Design: Getting the Professional Look*. London: Blueprint Publishing Ltd, 40 Bowling Green Lane, London EC1R 0NE

4 Further reading:

Ley P (1988) *Communicating with Patients*. London: Croom Helm, Chs 8 and 9

5 The Gobbledygook Test is reproduced by kind permission of the Plain English Campaign. See also:

Cutts M & Maher C (1980) *Writing Plain English: a Guide for Writers and Designers of Official Forms, Leaflets, Letters, Labels and Agreements*. Stockport: Plain English Campaign. Information and materials are available from: The Plain English Campaign, Outram House, 15 Canal St, Whaley Bridge, Stockport, SK12 7LS. Telephone: 0663 334541

6 For further information on non-sexist writing, see:

Miller C & Swift K (1981) *The Handbook of Non-Sexist Writing for Writers, Editors and Speakers*. London: The Women's Press.

7 For more about statistics, see:

Bayliss D (1983) Statistics for nurses 1: collection and presentation of data. *Nursing Times*, **79**, (43)

8 Published in booklet:

HEC (1982) *Beating Heart Disease*. London: Health Education Council. (Reproduced by kind permission of the Health Education Authority, London.)

9 Published in:

Patton A *et al* (1981) ABC of alcohol—nature of the problem. *British Medical Journal*, **283**, 1319. (Reproduced by kind permission of the Editor of the *British Medical Journal*)

10 Lung cancer data from:

Doll R & Peto R (1976) Mortality in relation to smoking . . . 20 years' observations in male British doctors. *British Medical Journal*. Published in the booklet *The Facts About Smoking—What Every Nurse Should Know* (1983) London: Health Education Council. (Reproduced by kind permission of the Editor of the British Medical Journal.)

11 Published in the booklet:

The Facts About Smoking—What Every Nurse Should Know (1983) London: Health Education Council. (Reproduced by kind permission of the Health Education Authority, London.)

12 Department of Transport (1990) *Drinking and Driving in Injury Road Accidents: The Facts*. Accident Fact Sheet 3/90. (Reproduced by permission of the Controller of HMSO.)

13 Published in:

Royal Society for the Prevention of Accidents (1983) *Home and Leisure Safety for Pre-retirement Course Organisers*. London: RoSPA. (Reproduced by kind permission of RoSPA)

Chapter 15 Working with the Mass Media

Summary

The chapter begins by identifying the key characteristics of the mass media and the variety of ways in which mass media are channels for health issues. This is followed by a discussion on what the mass media can be expected to achieve and how they can be used effectively. The chapter then concentrates on giving practical help to health promoters working with radio, television and the local press. There are exercises on preparing and presenting material on television and radio, and on writing a press release and a letter to the editor.

Health promoters are most likely to become involved with mass media when undertaking health promotion programmes or campaigns with the public, or when a health issue becomes a news item. You may also participate in the production of documentary programmes and articles, and probably most of your involvement will be with local newspapers and local radio. However, it is useful to put this into a wider context, and appreciate the range of ways by which health issues and messages are portrayed via the mass media.[1]

Mass Media as Channels for Health Issues

The mass media are channels of communication to large numbers of people: television, radio, magazines and newspapers, books, displays and exhibitions. Leaflets and posters are also mass media when they are used on a 'stand alone' basis, as opposed to use as a learning aid in face-to-face communication with an individual or a group. The key characteristics are the mass audience and that there is no, or little, interpersonal communication between the sender of the message and the mass audience: the message is sent through the media.

Health messages are sent through the mass media in a number of different ways:

- planned, deliberate health promotion, eg. displays and exhibitions on health themes,

Health Education Authority advertisements on television and in newspapers, Open University community education programmes on health;
- health promotion by advertisers and manufacturers of 'healthy' products and services, eg. advertisements for wholemeal bread or for toothpaste, educational leaflets on 'feeding your baby' or guides to 'healthy eating establishments' which also promote relevant products or services;
- books, documentaries and articles about health issues, eg. television programmes and magazines about food, AIDS, pollution or fitness;
- discussion of health issues as a by-product of news items or entertainment programmes, notably soap-opera series where a character has a health problem, such as being a victim of child sexual abuse or suffering from breast cancer;
- health (or anti-health) messages conveyed covertly or incidentally, eg. well-known personalities or fictional characters refusing cigarettes or, conversely, chain-smoking. The portrayal of alcohol on television, for example, conveys a norm of heavy drinking and associates consumption of alcohol with benefits rather than costs;[2]
- planned promotion of anti-health messages (probably denied or rationalised as not anti-health!), eg. advertisements for tobacco, sweets and chocolates;
- sponsorship of health-promoting events and services by organisations or commercial companies, such as sponsorship of sporting events by cigarette manufacturers or health promotion events by commercial companies. By associating with a health promoting event or service, the sponsor's product or service is brought to the public eye with an implied stamp of approval and a sense that it is somehow associated with health.

Using the Mass Media for Health Promotion

The fact that the message is sent via a medium (such as radio) makes it difficult to obtain immediate feedback and modify the communication to be responsive to the needs and characteristics of the audience. Audience phone-ins and exhibitions (although exhibitors may only involve a minority of people attending an exhibition) are a way of ensuring some two-way communication but the majority of communications are one-way.

This characteristic of one-way communication has major implications. For example, it is not possible for the sender to repeat, clarify or amplify the message so, in general, the mass media are best used for conveying simple rather than complex messages. Many research studies have now shown that the direct persuasive power of mass media is very limited.[3] Expectations that the mass media *alone* will produce dramatic long-term changes in health behaviour are doomed to disappointment. So it is important for you to know what kinds of success you can realistically expect when you use mass-media in your health promotion work.

Avoiding Pitfalls

Mass media messages must be carefully designed so that the right message gets to the target audience in a form appropriate to their needs and lifestyle. Commercial advertising applies in-depth research to the target audience; this has been applied in health promotion campaigns but it is obviously very costly.[4]

Health promotion using the mass media has the additional problem that the audience is often asked to identify with a message that they may find uncomfortable or even threatening (for example, messages about the threat of AIDS). The audience will search for rationalisations to reject the message, and one inaccurate detail in the portrayal of the lifestyle of the audience can result in rejection. This means that the images and scenarios require repeated testing on sample potential audiences.

Mass media campaigns can be an inappropriate response to many health problems. For example, a recent Department of Health mass media campaign costing £2 million directed at heroin misuse has been widely criticised.[5] Although it was very successful at penetrating the market (young people aged 13–20), and thus demonstrated the effectiveness of the mass media in raising awareness, it was most unlikely that it would have a large influence on drug-related behaviour. This was confirmed in the evaluation. The other influences on drug misuse such as unemployment, social deprivation, self-esteem, rebelliousness, curiosity, peer pressure, availability of drugs and beliefs about the gratifications provided, mean that this problem requires a much broader-based approach.

Using Mass Media Effectively

Mass media can be an effective element of planned programmes or campaigns when they are used to complement interpersonal approaches. They can also be used 'opportunistically' when events raise health issues in the news. But, in a nutshell, they are *most* effective when used to:

- set an agenda—for example, to raise consciousness about rubella as part of a vaccination campaign;
- deliver a simple message—for example, provide information about the availability of a screening service.

So it is evident that, properly used, the mass media can be a useful channel for health promotion, and we now look at this in more detail.

Achieving Health Promotion Aims

The following points summarise what we can reasonably expect to achieve, expressed in terms of the *health promotion aims* discussed in Chapter Six.

Raising health awareness. The mass media are very useful for drawing the attention of the public to a health issue, which then becomes a matter of public interest and debate. This is sometimes known as 'agenda-setting' because it raises the issues which are subsequently discussed, in the same way as a committee meeting agenda identifies the items for the committee's attention. Heart transplants and test-tube babies are examples of health issues which the news media put on the agenda of public debate. These examples also illustrate how the public agenda about health is usually actually about illness and disability, because most reporting of health issues stresses technological expertise and hospital-based curative medicine.[6] Positive health promotion is rarely hot news.

Increasing health knowledge. Once a topic is on the public agenda, the mass media can be used to inform the public and stimulate lively debate. Discussion about HIV testing, health service cuts, tobacco sponsorship of sports events and the provision of services for the disabled are examples of areas of informed debate on issues in the public eye in recent years.

Self-empowering and influencing attitude change, decision-making and behaviour change. It is not easy to identify the effect of the mass media in these areas, because mass media influences are inextricably bound up with all the other aspects of people's lives which affect their health attitudes and behaviour. However, it is clear that the mass media can be effective in eliciting an *immediate emotional response*, which may lead to an immediate action. An example of this is how people responded to the scare about brain damage caused by whooping cough vaccine by not taking their children to be vaccinated. Another example is the thousands of people who write for leaflets on how to give up smoking after a television programme on the subject. These are *short-term* responses. A permanent change in people's smoking, eating or drinking habits, for example, is unlikely to be achieved as a result of a mass media publicity alone.[7]

As the primary response of people to the mass media is emotional and not rational, it is very important not to raise anxieties irresponsibly. For example, publicity about rubella-damaged babies should always be accompanied by clear, simple and specific advice about the effects of rubella and how these can be avoided.

Deaths blamed on TV

Panorama distorted facts, says expert

By JOHN ILLMAN

BETWEEN 200 and 300 people died prematurely as a result of a TV programme, an eminent medical consultant claimed yesterday.

Dr Christopher Dallis said the BBC's controversial Panorama presentation on brain death in 1980 led to a sharp fall in the number of people prepared to donate their kidneys in the event of sudden death.

He accused the BBC of grossly distorting scientific data in the programme, adding: 'It had a tragic effect on the transplantation programme.'

Dr Pallis, consultant neurologist at London's Hammersmith Hospital, was speaking on Medical Disasters in Perspective at the British Association for the Advancement of Science meeting in Brighton.

Another speaker was Peter Goodchild, the BBC's head of science and features, whose subject was The Whys and Wherefores of The Reporting on So Called Disasters. But after he finished his lecture, Dr Pallis challenged him to explain the BBC's presentation of facts on the screen.

He maintained that matters apparently confirming brain death studies had been shown between quotation marks — but in fact the studies had not contained those statements. A BBC executive had said of this practice: 'We often put things in single quotes. That is our summary of what the text means. If it is a genuine quote it goes between double quotation marks.'

Asked if the BBC would continue to 'put things between quotation marks which are not quotes,' Mr Goodchild replied: 'I guess they probably will . . . but when you are quoting, it is normally quite clear, within the context of the programme, that double inverted commas means a quote. The point you are making about the programme is obviously a valid one. It has had a reaction.'

The mass media can be effective in eliciting an immediate emotional response (Reproduced from the *Daily Mail* of 27 August 1983 by the kind permission of Associated Newspapers Group.)

Effecting societal change. We have already said that the mass media are effective in raising health consciousness, increasing health knowledge and arousing an immediate emotional response. All these are important for producing a climate of public opinion which will favour societal change. An example of a societal change was the introduction in 1983 of legislation to enforce the wearing of car seat belts. This legislation was finally enacted after years of 'Clunk-click' media advertising and public debate, which *did not* in itself make people wear their seat belts in substantial numbers but helped to produce a climate of public opinion in which legislation was acceptable.[8]

The Mass Media as Part of an Overall Strategy

We have stressed that the mass media *alone* are unlikely to produce dramatic long-term changes in health behaviour; it is essential to realise that the most effective use of the mass media is as part of an overall strategy which includes face-to-face discussion and personal help.[9] For example, mass media publicity about sensible drinking should include information about where to go and who to see if people want help, and, of course, the helping agencies must be fully prepared to give that help.

The following example of a successful American mass media campaign illustrates the effectiveness of the mass media in agenda-setting and informing, and the importance of personal follow-up work by health professionals.

Example—The effective use of the mass media in health promotion

The Stanford University Heart Disease Prevention Programme[10]

This was an experiment in community behaviour change through education about the risks of cardiovascular disease, which was begun in 1972 in California.

The mass media elements involved exposing the population of the experimental communities to about three hours of television programmes, over fifty television announcements, one hundred radio spot broadcasts, several hours of radio programmes, weekly newspaper columns, newspaper advertisements and stories, posters in buses, stores and worksites, and printed material sent by mail to people's homes.

The research team found that the level of knowledge about risk factors associated with heart disease increased dramatically in the experimental communities and that there were accompanying reductions in saturated fat intake, cigarette smoking, plasma cholesterol levels, systolic blood pressure and the overall probability of contracting heart disease.

When the mass media elements were supplemented by face-to-face instruction not only were the results improved in the short term, but they were maintained over three years.

Creating Opportunities

Even though most health promoters are motivated to use the mass media, they may have misgivings and identify the need for further training.[11] For example, you may feel apprehensive about interviews with reporters from the local news media (local newspapers, radio and television). You may feel that 'They'll misquote me', 'I'll dry up if I'm interviewed', 'They'll sensationalise the issue' or 'I'll get into trouble with my manager'.

There may be more than a grain of truth in these fears, so what can be done to overcome them and make useful alliances with journalists? First, many health authorities and local authorities now employ public relations specialists with a background in journalism, and employees can enlist their help.[12]

Another way forward is to establish personal contact with local journalists. Do not wait for them to ring you—you ring them. Establish an informal, personal relationship:

get to know how they work and what their special areas of interest are, which will help to establish mutual trust and understanding. You can then approach them if you wish to give exposure to a particular topic, or if you wish to discuss how the media are portraying a current issue. The benefits are mutual; journalists will be more likely to approach you to get help with an item of health news.

Also, remember that it is in both your interests that you have good skills in communicating via the mass media, so why not ask for help with training needs? Many local radio and television journalists are happy to help with training. Short courses on using the media also may be available at local colleges and polytechnics.

Keep a record of what you find out about local media, and update it regularly. Include information on names and special interests of journalists and the 'copy dates' for each of the media in your area. The 'copy date' is the deadline for submitting written information ('copy'). For example, note the last day for submitting copy to a regular fortnightly magazine or local weekly paper. The daily newspapers should be able to respond immediately to a press release; radio often needs a few days to prepare coverage; television needs two weeks' advance notice to allow time for booking a film crew. This information will help you to be prepared when opportunities for useful media coverage arise.

The following sections give practical guidelines on working with radio, television and local newspapers. Possession of this information may also help in overcoming any fear of working with the news media.[13]

Working with Radio and Television

Using a spot on radio or television effectively requires research, preparation and skill. The following checklists have been prepared to help you to get your health promotion story to the right person and have the best chance of getting the coverage you want.

Researching Radio and TV

You need to listen to your local radio and watch television to see which programmes might be interested in your kind of news.

Basic information
- What hours do they broadcast?
- What region do they cover?
- Who is the audience? Does the profile alter according to the time of day?

The programmes
- What is covered on the news items?
- How many minutes of current affairs and local interest items?
- Are interviews used or straight reporting?
- What are the different kinds of programmes, and what is the proportion of time (news, current affairs, weekly events, phone-ins, music, etc).
- Which programmes use guests or 'experts'?
- Is there any local programme that regularly covers health issues?

- Is there a round-up of 'Events in the week ahead'—what is the deadline for information? How much detail do they give? What sort of events get covered?

Interviews

- Which programmes use interviews?
- For how many minutes do these last?
- What is the tone (bland, chatty, aggressive)?
- How long is the average answer before the next question? Time it!
- Are the interviews on location or in the studio?
- Are they recorded or live?
- Who are the presenters or interviewers on the programmes who might be interested in health? What is their style?

Finding Out About a Specific Programme

- What programme is it? What sort of approach does the programme have? How long is it? When is it to be transmitted? What kind of audience does it have?
- Why is your topic of interest *now*: is there some local or national controversy or news item which sparked off interest? If so, do you know all about it?
- How are you going to be presented: an information spot, an interview or a discussion panel?
  If it is an interview: who will do it? Will it be in the studio, or on location (perhaps in your workplace or outdoors), or 'down the line' (where you are in one studio and the interviewer in another)?
  If it is to be a discussion: who else will be taking part?
- Will it be broadcast live or recorded first?
- How much time are you likely to have on the programme?
- When and where is the broadcast or recording to take place?

Preparing the Message

- Do your homework. You may know a lot or a little about the subject, but in either case you need to identify exactly what it is you want to get across, and to have this very clearly in your mind *before* you are 'on the air'.
- Be positive. Emphasise the good news, *not* a series of don'ts. Tell people what they *can* do and emphasise the benefits.
- You should have two or three key points to put across, and *no more*. You can expand on these and describe them in different ways but do not overload your audience with too much detail or too many points. They will not remember the additional information anyway, and may even forget the key points.
- Use anecdotes and analogies to illustrate what you mean; simple messages do not have to be bald and boring. Tell stories (short ones!) and use real-life experiences. Put complex points over with everyday analogies, eg. 'Use too much fertiliser and you'll kill the plants—use the right amount and they'll grow strong and healthy. The same applies to food and people.'
- Avoid technical terms (unless these are essential, in which case use them and explain them) and jargon, but do not be patronising. It helps to pitch the level right if you

imagine that you are talking to an intelligent 14- to 15-year-old whom you have never met before.

Presenting Your Message

- Accept that you are nervous and regard it as a good thing because it means that you will be keyed up to do your best. Remember that the interviewer is there to help you tell your story and to put you at ease.
- Perform with more than 100% liveliness and conviction. Be alert and (if you are on television) look alert at all times. Always assume that the camera is on you even when you are not talking. Make sure your eyes look convincing and involved.
- Speak with your normal voice; if you have a regional accent this will make you more interesting to listen to. Speak clearly and distinctly, and (especially on radio) vary the pitch and speed.
- Make sure you say what *you* want to say. You do not have to follow the line of the interviewer's questions if, for good reason, you do not wish to. Provided you stick to the broad framework of agreed subjects, you have every right to steer the interview or discussion in such a way that you get over what you want to say. Regard the questions as springboards from which to make your points. For example, if you do not like a question you can say:

  'I can't really answer that question without explaining first that . . .'
  'The real problem behind all this is . . .'
  'We don't know the answer to that at the moment, but what we do know is . . .'

- When the interview is over, sit still, keep alert and keep quiet until you are *told* it is over.
- On television, wear what makes you feel comfortable and good. Avoid wearing blue or bright red, predominant stripes, small patterns or flashing jewellery. As you will appear as a 'talking head' for most of the time, pay special attention to what you wear in the neckline area.

Exercise—Looking good and sounding good on television and radio

1 Prepare you message

Select a health promotion topic that you are familiar with, eg. slimming, eating health-giving food, sensible drinking, feeding your baby, keeping fit, avoiding home accidents, living with stress.

Identify *three* key points you would want to put across in a five-minute radio or television interview. Be clear in your mind:

- what the three key points are;
- how you will explain them in an interesting way—what illustrations, analogies or anecdotes you could use;
- how you will develop your points further if you have time.

continued on next page

continued

2 Practise your presentation

Get a partner to act as your interviewer, and record your interview on an audio or a videotape. Ask a third person to be an observer. Play the tape back and assess your performance:

- did you sound/look lively, alert and convincing?
- was your voice clearly understandable? What did it sound like for speed and pitch?
- did you get your key points across? Did you do so in an interesting way?
- were you able to deal with 'difficult' questions?

Working with the Local Press

Local newspapers are an excellent medium for health promotion in a community. Local journalists will be interested in newsworthy health issues and it is worth studying the newspapers to see who writes about health topics. This is a checklist of what to look for when researching a paper.

Basic information

- When is it published?
- What are the deadlines for copy?
- What locality does it cover?
- How many readers and who are they?

The copy

- What is the style (bright, sober, campaigning, etc.)?
- What is the average length of articles (often different for news, business, features)?
- What percentage of articles have photographs?
- How many photographs per page?
- How are photographs used generally?
- How are quotations used?

The subjects

- What sorts of stories are used (local, jolly, controversial, educational) and how are they treated?
- What is the ratio of coverage for news: features; business; diary, etc.?
- How long and how full is the 'events ahead' section?
- Are there special sections or supplements on health, education, women, etc.? How long and on what day?
- Are there regular columnists? What are their special interests?

The language

- What is the average length of sentences?
- What is the average length of paragraphs?

- What kind of language is used (multisyllabic, slangy, turgid, lively, short and simple)?

Your special interests

- Anything in the papers that may be of special use to you or to your organisation?

This may seem a lot to cope with, especially if you have a number of local and regional newspapers. Gradually build up expertise, with a fact sheet on each one. This will be indispensable for targeting your press releases.

EVENING POST, THURSDAY, MARCH 2, 1989 — 11

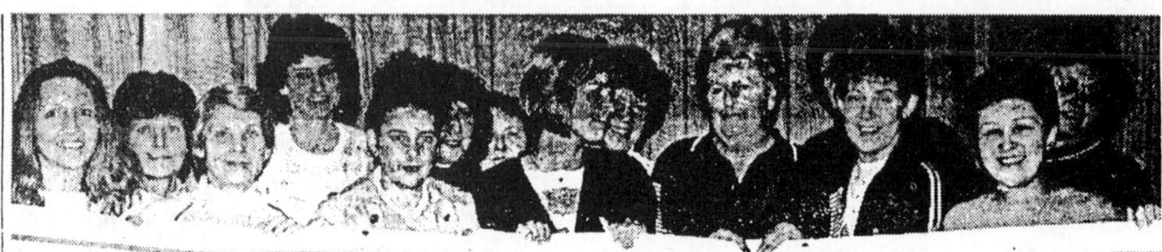

National No SMOKING DAY

Wednesday March 8th

HELPING PEOPLE WHO WANT TO STOP SMOKING

Quit and get fit . . . women at the YMCA in Totterdown, Bristol, join the campaign to stop smoking

QUIT — BUT DON'T RUN OUT OF PUFF

By Kevan Blackadder

SMOKERS wanting to give up on National No Smoking Day will be given every encouragement by a new group, a councillor and 22 keep-fit women.

The Smoking Prevention Field Support Project was launched this week at the Redland faculty of Bristol Polytechnic.

The unit, which receives a £120,000 grant from the health education authority, aims to raise the profile of smoking prevention work, both locally and nationally.

It has already worked to discourage young women from smoking, for tighter controls on tobacco advertising, and campaigned for more smoke-free areas in public places.

And it will be closely involved with National No Smoking Day next Wednesday, which will see the deputy leader of Bristol City Council start his attempt to give up.

Councillor Jack Fisk is backing the council's desire for at least one smoker in each department to give up by joining in himself.

And at Totterdown YMCA, 22 women have signed up for the latest Quit and Get Fit course.

The course, first run at Totterdown, is now held at 50 centres nationwide.

It includes an exercise programme to get the lungs and heart working without a constant input of smoke.

The theme for this year's day is "Break Free — Plant a Tree" because one tree every fortnight has to be cut down to provide the tobacco leaf for the average smoker.

It is estimated that five million hectares are cleared of trees each year for smokers.

The council staff will be sponsored to give up smoking and hope to raise enough money to plant 20 trees in a city park.

Local News is Local People (Reproduced with kind permission of the Editor, *Bristol Evening Post*).

How to Write a Press Release[14]

To write a press release (sometimes also called a 'news release') you will need:

- A good text—use a title to grab attention. The guts of the story must be in the first short paragraph. However complex the subject there will be one outstanding thing which makes it newsworthy. Start with a bang by spelling this out. Make your points in order of importance (a story gets cut from the bottom up). Use short sentences and easy language, with no abbreviations or jargon. Using quotations can bring a piece to life. Don't be afraid of making up things which you or your group might have said (check first with the people concerned). For example, 'Mrs Gloria Slim, the District Dietitian, said "I am delighted at the number of hospitals which now offer patients a choice of vegetarian and traditional ethnic dishes on the menu".'
- A short text—keep it brief, to one page if possible. If longer, type 'More follows . . .' at the bottom right hand corner. Don't carry over paragraphs or sentences to the next page. Type 'Ends' after the last line of the release. Sentences must be short, paragraphs brief.
- A local angle for a local paper—news is people and local news is local people. So focus on people rather than making generalised statements or quoting dry statistics. For example, say: 'Last week three Bloggsville children were admitted to the Royal Infirmary after accidentally swallowing weedkiller. This brings to over 100 the number of children who have been accidentally poisoned this year. Sister Florence Nightingale, in charge of the Accident and Emergency Department, said: "It is heartbreaking to see the needless distress this causes . . .".'
- Good timing—your news will not be newsworthy on the day of election of a new prime minister! Yesterday's news is dead, today's may still be of interest, but tomorrow's has the best chance of being printed. Alert newspapers a few days in advance so that they can send reporters to cover an interesting event. For example, contact on a Friday or Monday is usually best for a weekly paper published on the following Friday. If you want to launch a story at a particular time, use the 'embargo' system. This means writing, for example, 'Not for use until Wednesday July 3rd 1991' or 'Embargoed 6 pm July 3rd 1991' across the top of the press release.
- Good presentation—A4 paper, headed with a logo if possible. Colour catches the eye, so a coloured heading or coloured paper will make your release stand out.
- Good technique—journalists work at speed, so make their task easier by
  - —using only one side of the page, placing the text centrally on the page
  - —using a layout with double spacing
  - —leaving at least one inch (2–3 cm) margin on either side
  - —putting a release date or embargo date at the top
  - —giving names and telephone numbers of people in your organisation for further information (including an after-hours telephone number)
  - —sending it to a named journalist, if possible
  - —not underlining any words (because this gives printers instructions to use italics).
- A big photograph—if you are sending one, 7″ × 5″ or 10″ × 8″, generally black and

white are preferred, with a full label on the back giving names and details. Don't forget to include the names of everyone in the picture ('The picture shows left to right June Bloggs and Sam Smith . . .') and explain what they are doing ('presenting Healthy Eating awards at 3 pm on Tuesday March 10th at Bloggsville Town Hall'). Never *write* on the back of a photograph, as this will destroy the quality. Photos should be eye-catching and clear.

- Good communication—send a copy of the press release to everyone who will be affected, including your organisation's press officer, and to everyone mentioned or otherwise involved in the story.
- A final check—before you send it, ask yourself if this would tell you:
  What?
  Who?
  When?
  Where?
  Why?
  How?

Example—Press release

KOFFCOUNTY DISTRICT HEALTH AUTHORITY

PRESS RELEASE 1st October 1991

SMOKERS HOTLINE LAUNCHED

Koffcounty's Smokers Hotline got off to a flying start this week, when Dr Jo Goodheart, a specialist in heart disease at Kofftown General Hospital, launched the service.

The hotline has been set up as part of Koffcounty Heart Week (2nd–9th October), to help people who want to stop smoking. All those ringing Kofftown 112233 will be sent a free pack of useful ideas to help them give up, including tips from ex-smokers and information about local stop-smoking groups.

'I smoked myself when I was younger and I remember what a struggle I had to stop. Many of my patients with heart trouble also find it incredibly difficult,' said Dr Goodheart. 'That's why I'm delighted to launch this scheme. The pack has lots of useful information to help people over the difficulties.'

continued on next page

continued

Smokers have a two to three times greater risk of having a heart attack than non-smokers. At least 80 per cent of heart attacks in men under 45 are thought to be due to cigarette smoking. Stopping smoking could lead to 150 fewer deaths each year of men and women under 65 in Koffcounty.

ENDS

For further information, please contact:

Sally Prohealth

Senior Health Promotion Officer

Central Health Clinic,

People's Lane,

Kofftown KT1 2YZ

Telephone Kofftown 456789 (day) or Nextown 123456 (evenings)

Writing Letters to the Editor

Another way of using the local paper as a medium for health promotion is by writing letters to the editor. This can keep an issue in the public eye for some time, and provides good opportunities for public debate of controversial issues. Letters to the editor should be short (some newspapers restrict length), to the point and be on one topic only.

Exercise—Writing for the local paper

1. Write a press release about a health promotion issue you are currently concerned about (for example, school meals, uptake of antenatal classes, glue-sniffing or the local accident black spot).
2. Write a letter to the editor supporting a current health education campaign, or drawing attention to a specific need for health promotion.

Notes, References and Further Reading

1 For general background reading on the role of the mass media in relation to health promotion, see:

McCron R & Budd J (1987) Mass communication and health education. In: *Health Education: Perspectives and Choices* (ed I Sutherland). Cambridge: National Extension College

Leathar D S, Hastings G B & Davies J K (eds) (1986) *Health Education and the Media*. Oxford: Pergamon Press

2 Hansen A (1986) The portrayal of alcohol on television. *Health Education Journal*, **45**, 127–31

Institute for Alcohol Studies (1985) *The Presentation of Alcohol in the Mass Media*. Report of a Seminar, January 1985. Institute for Alcohol Studies, 12 Caxton Street, London

3 For a review of the research, see:

Tones K, Tilford S & Robinson Y (1990) *Health Education: Effectiveness and Efficiency*. London: Chapman & Hall, Ch 6

4 Player D A & Leathar D S (1981) Developing socially sensitive advertising. In Leathar D S, Hastings G B & Davies J K (eds) *Health Education and the Media*. Oxford: Pergamon Press, 187–198

5 See, for example:

Tones B K (1986) Preventing drug misuse: the case for breadth, balance and coherence. *Health Education Journal*, **45**, 223–30

6 Best G, Dennis J & Draper P (1977) *Health, the Mass Media and the National Health Service*. London: Unit for the Study of Health Policy

7 For example, see:

Raw M & Van de Pligt (1981) Can television help people stop smoking? In Leathar D S, Hastings G B & Davies J K (eds) *Health Education and the Media*. Oxford: Pergamon Press, 387–398

8 Dillow I, Swann C & Cliff K S (1981) A study of the effect of a health education programme in promoting seat-belt wearing. *Health Education Journal*, **40**(1), 14

In 1981, Parliament agreed in principle to the compulsory wearing of seat belts. In 1983, regulations came into force: *Motor Vehicles (Wearing of Seat Belts) Regulations* 1982 S.I. no. 1203

9 For example, the complementary use of different media and methods—television programmes complementing school-based education and parental involvement—is discussed in:

Flay B R *et al* (1987) Implementation effectiveness trial of a social influences smoking prevention programme using schools and television. *Health Education Research*, **2**, 385–400.

Open learning programmes which use media such as written texts, video and audiotapes, in combination with peer-group support networks, tutorials, tutor assessment and workshops, are a good example of using complementary methods and media.

10 Maccoby N & Solomon D (1981) Experiments in risk reduction through community health education. In Meyer M (ed) *Health Education by Television and Radio*. Munich: K G Saur Verlag, 140–166

11 Flora J A & Wallack L (1990) Health promotion and mass media use: translating research into practice. *Health Education Research*, **5**, 73–80

12 A useful book on using the media produced for health workers is:

South East Thames Regional Health Promotion Group (1985) *Getting Through*. South East Thames Regional Health Authority, Thrift House, Collington Avenue, Bexhill-on-Sea, East Sussex TN39 3NQ

13 For a basic, practical guide to all aspects of public relations, including dealing with press, radio and TV, developing campaigns and publicity stunts, see:

McIntosh D & McIntosh A (1985) *A Basic PR Guide for Charities*. Directory of Social Change. Available from: Community Education Development Centre, Lyng Hall, Blackberry Lane, Coventry CV2 3JS. Telephone: 0203 638660

For help with putting messages over effectively, using a variety of media, see:

Zeitlyn J (1988) *Getting Your Message Across*. Interchange Books. Available from Community Education Development Centre, address above

14 This section is based partly on:

Association of Community Workers (1986) *Talking Point*, **74** (June) 1–4, Association of Community Workers, Colombo Street Sports & Community Centre, 25 Colombo Street, London SE1 8DP

Index

action plans 98–9, 166, 201–2
adult education 156, 175–89
advocacy 154, 170, 191, 195
agendas
  committees, of 108
  groups, of 150
  hidden 145–6
  setting 245
agents and agencies, of health promotion 48–56
AIDS, policies on 215, 217, 224
aims and methods of health promotion 90–1, 93
aims
  hierarchy of 86
  aims, setting 32–8, 76–7, 86–90
  health promotion approaches to 167, 169–70
  policies on 217–8, 224
assertiveness training 91
attitude change 91, 96, 159, 172, 204

behaviour change 91, 96, 140, 166–72
  approach 36, 37
  strategies for 166–72
beliefs 162–4
body language *see* non-verbal communication
brainstorming 151
buzz groups 152

campaigns 91, 219–20
choice 158–74
  informed 37
client-centred 121–4
  approach 36, 37
codes of practice 25, 44–5
commercial organisations 25, 51
committees 107–8
communication barriers 124–6
communication skills 110–2, 124–37
community
  work based in 91, 192–205
  definition of 191
  development 39, 196–9
  health projects 199–204
  work 191, 204–5
Community Health Council (CHC) 43, 54
Community Health Initiatives Resource Unit (CHIRU) 18, 206
competence 27
competences, see health promotion competences
conflict resolution styles 109–10
consumerism 71
co-ordination 104–6
coping strategies 168–9
counselling 165–6
  in groups 140

dietitians 54
discussion leading 150–2
displays 226, 233–4
district health authorities *see* health authorities
district nursing teams 53
drug education 50

economic activities 25, 26
economic conditions *see* socio-economic conditions
education approach 36 *see also* health promotion approaches
effectiveness and efficiency 101
employment training 51
empowerment *see* self-empowerment

English National Board for Nursing 53, 60
environmental
  change 12
  conditions 13
  measures 25–6
  health officers 43, 55
ethics 32
ethical decisions 42–4
  issues in health promotion 33–42
ethnic backgrounds 126
epidemiological data 73
European Community 50
evaluation 94–8
  key terms 101
  of outcomes 96–7
  of processes 97–8
example, learning by 171
experimental learning 159
expressed need 68–9

facilitation 28, 36, 192
  of groups 140, 141–2
Family Health Services Authorities
  (FHSA's) 52–3
feelings
  objectives concerned with 89
  reflecting 133
felt need 68
fiscal measures 25
food
  manufacturers 51
  policies 225
  politics of 223
force field analysis 58, 212
framework, of areas of health promotion
  activity 26

games in group work 149, 162
general practitioners 53
goals of health promotion 87, 90–1
government departments 50
green movement 13, 18
group
  dynamics 144
  work, definition of 139
groups
  leadership of 140–4
  purposes of 140
  self-help *see* self-help groups
  setting up 146–8
  skills 139

health
  authorities 52
  boards 52
  definitions of 6, 8
  dimensions of 6–8
  determinants of 9–14
  inequalities in *see* inequalities in health
  information 41, 72–5
  targets 13, 87, 209
  visitors 54
Health and Safety Executive 51, 216
Health Education Authority 52, 59
Health Education Board for Scotland 52, 59
health education
  certificate courses 57, 61
  definition of 20
  objectives of 88–9
  primary, secondary and tertiary 24
  in schools *see* school health education
  in adult education *see* adult education
Health For All
  movement 13
  network 213, 223
  targets 13
health promotion
  activities 20–6
  agents and agencies 48–56
  aims and methods of 91
  approaches to 35–8
  competences 27–9
  definition of 19–20
  glossary 30
  goals of 32–8, 86–92
  and health education 20
  models of 32, 35–8
  objectives of 87
  officers 52–3
  planning 84–100
  policies 215–9
  priorities 78–80
  workplace, in the 216–9
healthy cities network 13, 17 *see also* Health
  For All network
healthy eating, goals and methods of 93
healthy public policies, *see* public policies,
  healthy
higher education, institutions of 55–6
housing 10–2
humanistic psychology 172

immunisation 24
inequalities in health 10, 11, 13, 39, 192–3
influencing, policies 210–5
information
  finding & using 72–5
  statistical 237–40
  systems 113
Institution of Environmental Health
  Officers 64
instructions, giving 183–6

language barriers 126–7
leadership styles 140–3
leaflets 226, 229, 232, 234
learning, experimental *see* experimental
  learning 175–7
legislation 25
lifestyles 12, 17, 20, 33, 36
listening skills 130–4
local authorities 54–5
local education authorities 55

management
  definition of 103
  of health promotion 103–20
  of stress 118
  of time 113–6
  of voluntary organisations 116
marketing 28, 71–2, 81
  definition of 71–2
mass media 243–56
  advertising 244
medical approach 35–7
meetings of committees *see* committees
  participating in 106–7
midwives 54
models *see* health promotion, models of
morbidity and mortality data 73

National Health Service (NHS) 52–4
  NHS Training Directorate 52, 59
need, comparative 69
  concepts of 68–9
  expressed 68
  felt 68
  normative 68
needs
  identifying 70–1
  of service users 71–2
network, informal 48, 49, 56
networking 28, 194, 202, 213
new public health movement 13, 25
non-verbal communication 127–31
Northern Ireland Health Promotion
  Unit 52, 59

objectives
  educational 88–9
  setting 86–90
occupational health services 49, 56
Open University 55, 61–2
organisational development 22, 25–6
organisations
  commercial *see* commercial organisations
  national 50–4
  local 54–6
  religious 52

paperwork, managing 113
patient education 183–6, 188
persuasion 35–7
pharmacists 54
planning 84–102
police officers 56
policies, health promotion 28, 215–9
political
  action 13, 20, 25, 214
  change 193, 210–1
  influencing 212–5
positive health
  activities 23–5
posters 229
practice nurses 53
press releases 253–5
preventive health services 24, 26
primary care facilitators 54
primary health care 59
  teams 53–4
professional associations 51, 210
professionalisation 41
priorities 78–80
prison officers 56
probation officers 56
Public Health Alliance 17
public health medicine 82
  faculty of 17
public health, new, *see* new public health
  movement
public policies 208–11
  healthy 13, 25, 209
public speaking 180–3

questioning 134–7
questionnaire design 74, 82, 96, 97

racism 33, 126, 236
radio 248–51
readability tests 234–5
recreation officers 55
rehabilitation programmes 24
relaxation 143–4
report writing 111–2
research methods 101–2
resources for health promotion 92, 94, 148,
  229–236
risk factors 73
role play 161, 185–6
rounds 151
Royal Society for the Prevention of
  Accidents (RoSPA) 49

self-empowerment 19, 36, 37, 41, 46, 142,
  159–66, 170
self-esteem 159

self governing hospitals 52
self-help groups 140, 191
self-monitoring 167
sexism 12, 236–8
smoking policies 215, 223–4
social services staff 55
societal change
  approach 36, 37
socio-economic conditions 11, 13, 32–3, 36–7, 39, 44
socio-economic data 73–4
sponsorship 41
statistics 237–240
stress management *see* management of stress
surveys 74, 82, 97, 102

targets, for Health For All *see* Health For All targets
teaching 175–89
teamwork 105–6
television 51, 248–51
The Advisory Council on Alcohol and Drug Education (TACADE) 61
The Training Agency 49, 50–1
time management *see* management of time
trade unions 51
training, in health promotion 57–8
Training and Enterprise Councils (TECs) 49, 52

unemployment 11

values 35–8
  clarifying 159–64
victim-blaming 12, 17, 20
voluntary organisations 49, 51
  management of *see* management of voluntary organisations

workplace, health promotion in *see* health promotion in the workplace policies
World Health Organisation 13, 17, 19, 20, 29, 49, 50, 53, 59
  definitions of health 6, 8, 20
written materials 229, 232–8

youth groups 49, 55